A Love Affair With Cancer

JOHN W. PATTISON

Bloomington, IN   Milton Keynes, UK
authorHOUSE

AuthorHouse™
1663 Liberty Drive, Suite 200
Bloomington, IN 47403
www.authorhouse.com
Phone: 1-800-839-8640

AuthorHouse™ UK Ltd.
500 Avebury Boulevard
Central Milton Keynes, MK9 2BE
www.authorhouse.co.uk
Phone: 08001974150

This book is a work of non-fiction. Unless otherwise noted, the author and the publisher make no explicit guarantees as to the accuracy of the information contained in this book and in some cases, names of people and places have been altered to protect their privacy.

First published by AuthorHouse 7/3/2006

ISBN: 1-4259-1212-5 (sc)

Printed in the United States of America
Bloomington, Indiana

This book is printed on acid-free paper.

Special Thanks

I would like to say a sincere thank you to the following:

Mathew Wright, my newfound friend, for your words of wisdom and reflection. Like me, you have an appreciation and enthusiasm for life, but also a devotion to the Hawks. I value and look forward to our continued friendship.

My family, who without exception supported me when I was most vulnerable.

Keith Barton and Mr. Dibbs, it was an honour and privilege to play together with you guys (or an attempt to in my case) and I will cherish those memories forever. We truly are 'Spirits of the Age'. You helped take my 'space rock' experience to new heights and I will always be indebted.

And also thanks to life itself, you are something special and I love you. I could not have written this book without you.

To anyone and everyone who has been part of my life, you know who you are and I thank you.

Supported by an unrestricted educational grant from Ortho Biotech.

Foreword

I was thrilled and honoured when my friend John Pattison asked me, quite meekly, if I'd be prepared to write a foreword to his life story. When he told me, he was calling his autobiography *A Love Affair With Cancer* I have to admit I was intrigued, too.

I knew a little of John's story and a little more about the ravaging effects of cancer from friends, loved ones and relatives and simply couldn't understand how or why anyone could ever have a "love affair" with such an appalling disease.

But then I didn't know *all* of John's story. I hadn't read it - it was still being written at the time - but now I have I do understand. And understanding a little about cancer, about the fact that no two people ever have the same experience; about how it haunts its victims not just before and during treatment but afterwards as well. I think that's important information for all of us to know.

I've lost my father and grandfather to bowel cancer. My two uncles have it at the moment. I nursed a beautiful young woman through breast cancer. I only wish I had read John's book before doctors broke the news to Dad or told Caroline the lump in her breast was indeed malignant. I'd have been a lot more use I'm sure.

The facts concerning cancer are horrible. I do a lot of talks about the Big C. To gain the audience's attention I tell them that if the person on their left doesn't develop cancer and the person on the right is also destined to have a cancer-free life then they themselves will probably develop the disease. That's what the statistics tell us.

But John's book tells us an awful lot more. A cancer diagnosis doesn't spell the end. A failed treatment course doesn't mean a life is over. *A Love Affair with Cancer* shows how hope, love, care and devotion can change the course of someone's life, bringing light where there was only darkness before, hope where there was none.

I sincerely hope you read this book – and find it as inspiring as I do. Have a long, happy and fulfilling life.

Matthew Wright
Television presenter.

Introduction

The moment that changed my personal future and indeed the rest of my life took place within the confines of a busy cancer ward at Newcastle General Hospital way back in 1976, even though the real story had begun one year earlier. At that time (1976), I was completely demoralised by the ravages of cancer and its unforgiving treatment. I had been receiving treatment on and off for more than a year and yet despite that, it had proved unsuccessful, so now my mind was made up, enough was enough. Weak, tearful and ready to accept defeat, I could take no more. My feeling was that there was only so much one person could take and I simply could take no more of the treatment, whatever the consequences!

I had already endured many months of the unrelenting ravages of chemotherapy and now I'm told that the cancer is progressing despite all of that ferocious treatment that had gone before. During chemotherapy, I had struggled both mentally and physically to deal with the persistent barrage of side effects and my inability to accept the uncertainty that is a cancer diagnosis and so, the time had come to accept the consequences of a body gripped by cancer and which was unwilling to release its deathly hold. My decision? To accept no further treatment, whatever the outcome may be and at that moment in time, I knew what that outcome would be, yet that was my decision and strangely I was relieved at having mustered the courage to make that choice.

It wasn't just the physical destruction caused by a malignancy that I objected to, it was the fact that it was eating into my very soul, sowing seeds of doubt within my mind, interfering with every element of my very existence. Slowly but surely, it was leaving a permanent and unseen reminder, a hidden scar and a legacy, which if I were fortunate enough to survive, would last forever.

So, the confrontation between me, an immature and terrified teenager and a young, and perhaps out of his depth Staff Nurse (Sid) proved a pivotal moment of decisive change and a defining instance in my life, a moment that was destined to happen, a consequence of fate. And so, when as a young and angry, confused and obstinate cancer patient, I set my mind to something then it would be a brave nurse who attempted to interject and change that decision, no matter how well intentioned those actions were.

However, with compassion, empathy and a dogged determination not to stand back and watch me throw my life away, Sid did exactly that, interjected. During what seemed an eternity, Sid told me what I already knew, *"without treatment I would die"*, then he listened to my counterargument and I again listened to him. His support and persuasion worked, and he reversed my decision not to have more treatment, his fervent optimism was admirable and yet he did not glory in his success.

Had he not been there, the story would have ended here .... However, he was and it turned out to be just the start of a lifelong cancer journey that would take me through many new and unknown dimensions in my life, as it would turn out my association with cancer would be a lifelong relationship. Today, thirty years later it continues to be a significant component in my life, without doubt, *'A Love Affair with Cancer'*.

Chapter One

Personal emotions do not follow a pre-arranged script when attacked by the turmoil of malignant disease. The confusion inflicted on the mind and the desire to rid the body of its unwanted accomplice is one of the hardest issues to confront.

World Of Tiers

Fundamentally, the real story begins in 1957 when I was born to Ruby and John Walker Pattison in South Shields, a small seaside town nestling on the North East coast. My father was a well-respected Plumber working along the banks of the River Tyne in South Shields and my mam came from a large family of five other sisters and one brother. I have one younger sister Allyson and, my childhood was, in my opinion, uneventful but happy. As a youngster, I enjoyed all that a normal child would, such as finding trouble, football and especially fishing. As a teenager, I had a good circle of friends, both at school and socially. Meanwhile, Newcastle United had been a passion of mine since Uncle Glynn took me along to my first match way back in 1969 and like most schoolboys I had always dreamed of playing football for the black and white magpies. However and realistically, most of the other lads at school were much better at the game than I would ever be. Yes, I had played a handful of games for the school football team, Chuter Ede, but more often than not I'd be on the touchline as the substitute and despite my eagerness to play and watch football at that early age, even Newcastle United would not be able to compete with my real passion, music. But, not just any music, music that would affect my inner soul and influence the rest of my life, music that would prove to be a driving force of motivation.

I would describe myself as an animated extrovert, easy going with an opinion on most things, as most people do. I'm easy to get on with, relaxed and I like to think that I respect the views and opinions of others. I am very proud of my family and also my hometown, South Shields. During those early years music became my obsession, it was the focus of my attention to the exclusion of most other things including my education; it was the centre of my universe.

At the tender age of fifteen (1971) and while still at school I discovered a band that was, in many respects still in their infancy regarding their own development. The band, called Hawkwind, formed in the late 60's by former street busker, Dave Brock, they played what was described as 'space rock' and I immediately identified with it. A raw mixture of stunning light shows, electronics, rhythm guitar, saxophone and percussion, an almost Neanderthal approach to music which has influenced the way so many other bands deliver their music and continues to influence music even today. Now, to call it Neanderthal is not an insult to Hawkwind, it's just that they were in an ascendancy of their own discovery at that particular time. Meanwhile, Hawkwind played many venues the length and breadth of the country and many of these concerts were free shows, often supporting worthy charitable causes. Sadly for me however, a young fifteen year old, I had to be content with their records and the ever present scripting in the national media, mainly Sounds and Melody Maker magazines. I was not, at that particular juncture in time to realize just how influential and motivational the band would become, how they would unknowingly support me through a psychological battle unlike any other and how they would continue to influence my life, even to this day.

By my own admission I did not take school as seriously as I should have, instead treating it as one huge adventure. Life was a joke and I could be the world's greatest practical joker, while my best friend at that moment in time, Alan Robertson, known as Robbo was equally as mad as I was. In fact, our mutual friends and classmates would often cringe with fear when Robbo and I were together and preparing to act out some churlish tomfoolery on another unsuspecting friend.

To use a common reference, I considered and acknowledged myself as 'daft as a brush'. Even to this day, I enjoy a good practical joke and let's face it, you can't be serious all day, light-hearted joking is an extremely important component of life. Humour and laughter are incredible assets; they help to keep your feet firmly on the ground, but also to ensure that as a person, you remain sober minded in light of the pressures of every day life and life can certainly produce pressure as I was soon to discover!

Robbo and I both enjoyed our rock music and like so many, it was always our intention to become rock stars and true to this lifestyle I had been letting my hair grow for some time, this would be my statement, my identity, my freedom. Robbo and I would spend hours upon hours at each other's houses listening to music. When we weren't at home listening to music, we'd be in the second hand record shops selling albums to buy others, for me though; I had my collection of Hawkwind vinyl and would never part with these, they were my prized possessions, as valuable as gold. However, unlike me, Robbo preferred the softer tones of Roxy Music in comparison to my personal preference, the innovative and imaginative Hawkwind.

Into 1972 and life was all about rock music for me. At night, five or six of us would meet up after school and quite innocently walk the streets listening to good music on an old-fashioned cassette player. It was harmless entertainment and I suppose you could argue, it kept us out of trouble. Thursday and Friday nights were youth club nights. At St Hilda's most Friday nights, there would be a disco and occasionally a live band. The youth club was an excellent place to socialise, but the good thing about these discos was that around 9 o'clock the DJ would play a rock slot with around half a dozen well established rock tracks, such as Deep Purple, Black Sabbath, Led Zeppelin and the like. However, occasionally I would convince the disc jockey to play a Hawkwind track, when they did, it would most often be, not surprisingly, Silver Machine, and as you would expect, I was always the first to get onto the floor to do my stuff. Silver Machine had been a huge chart success for the band, peaking at number three in the music charts.

Most often than not there would only be a couple of us who would venture onto the dance floor during the rock session, although occasionally, a couple of the girls might also join us, but purely for the purpose of ridicule. However, nothing would have stopped me dancing once Hawkwind was playing as I saw my attempts at artistic impression a tribute to the band I now revered. It was at this moment in time that I met Dave, a dedicated Status Quo fan and he also felt that when his band played, he should be there on the dance floor. Subsequently, each Friday, once the rock session was underway we would seek each other out as if we had a secret mission to accomplish. Dave and I became great friends, in fact, he became a lifelong dependable friend and I was honoured to be his best man, not once but twice. At the third attempt of marriage, he wisely chose someone else to undertake the duty and he remains happily married to this day to Lyn, he also remains a good and close friend.

I could recall many anecdotal stories about those early days and the mischief I regularly found myself in, most often of course I didn't have to look far for it, trouble seemed as though it could find me quite easily. However, I'll leave that for another day. This book is intended to be an insight into my difficulties and dilemmas when facing the most difficult challenge known to man, the fight against cancer. However, my story is different to many others because it did not just continue to be my fight, as you will discover later.

Importantly, this chronicle is not about how individuals should respond to a cancer diagnosis, nor is it intended to be a prescriptive guide to coping with the emotional imposition suffered when cancer is diagnosed. Yet, in writing this book I have found a catharsis, which I sincerely hope, may help others who have been touched in some way, shape or form by the condition which medical science still has little answer for. Naturally, we all respond in different ways to the pressure and emotions, the fears and stigma that this disease can elicit and no textbook can tell you what the correct response is, and which is not. Cancer is a condition that has affected probably every man, woman and child in the country to some degree, whether it is a friend, relative or you individually. 'A Love Affair with Cancer' is my own personal story, my journal of events and coping strategies, the high's and the many low's of my cancer trajectory and undoubtedly, it will be very different to every other individual that has ever had or been touched by cancer. There are no correct or incorrect responses to the bombshell that is brought about by a cancer diagnosis, it is very much an individual response and without doubt, it will initiate a whole myriad of different instinctive responses in each and every person that is diagnosed.

Personal emotions do not follow a pre-arranged script when attacked by the turmoil of malignant disease. The confusion inflicted on the mind and, the desire to rid the body of its unwanted accomplice is one of the hardest issues to confront. The feelings of helplessness and despair are at times almost constant companions, yet at other times the pleasure and sanctity of life give you an unexpected determination to battle on. The fear and emotional retribution cancer brought gave me an appreciation of life generally, although it took me some time to realise how sweet and important life truly was and remains. Cancer has not only influenced my views and opinions on life generally, it makes me the person I am today, without that diagnosis and subsequent treatment, what my life would have been no one will ever know.

It would be wrong not to pay tribute and to acknowledge the love that I received from my family, especially mum, dad and my dear sister Allyson. However, as you will soon realise, another dimension was specifically inspirational and played a significant role in my recovery. In many respects, the cancer diagnosis allowed me to discover myself and to appreciate the wonders of each and every day, but there were times when I would resent life itself.

My life experiences, particularly the trauma of fighting tooth and nail to beat the demon that is cancer, have made me who I am today. But, without divulging too soon in this biography the secrets and the anxieties that have plagued my life and there have been many, and so much more than my individual fight against cancer, much more that has allowed me to discover myself. My life to date has, at times been difficult, although it has always been a pleasure of surprising discovery and I would not, in hindsight, change any of it, well perhaps a couple of things, like a failed marriage. I certainly feel fortunate the way my life has been mapped out by fate, and my experiences to date have allowed me to appreciate all that is good and worthwhile in life itself. I could not envisage my current status in any other shape.

Cancer has played a significant part in my life, it has made me who I am and for that I am appreciative. Now this may sound like an unusual thing to say having been ravaged and unceremoniously attacked by an invisible disease and apparently taken fairly close to death on more than one occasion and so what am I grateful for? Well, it's the ability to reflect on those past years, to understand who I am and what is and what is not important in my life, to appreciate the difficulty other individuals face and being able as so many do, to overcome adversity and to look forward to tomorrow.

This is my story and how I dealt with the affects of not only the disease and its treatments, but also its long-term effects and how I deal with the permanent legacy of malignancy. It is also about the harrowing and difficult dilemma I faced as a father being told that my daughter had terminal leukaemia. Cancer has given me a virtue that I firmly believe would have been absent had it not touched my very existence and threatened it more than once.

So many people today take life for granted and yet it is a privilege for all of us to be part of it. Life and health is not an entity that you can place a price upon; it is invaluable and also precious and deserves to be respected. How and why we are who we are, no one really knows and it is the ultimate question that I could not possibly give any definitive answers too, no one can. I can of course offer an opinion; an opinion influenced by the way cancer has affected my life and my family. Moreover, being affected by cancer certainly influences your approach to life, your philosophical beliefs and all that you as an individual represent and believe, so in that respect, I am like all other cancer patients, reflective, philosophical, grateful and respectful of a condition that society fears more than any other. The difference is that not everyone affected by cancer will come up with the same answers; all of us, whether a patient, parent, partner or significant other will have a differing perspective on the many perplexing challenges that life can throw at us and that cancer can throw at us, the numerous dilemmas we face and that are instigated by a cancer diagnosis. Significantly, I believe it is cancer that influences those opinions; at least it was in my situation.

Each of the chapters in my book have been given a specific title; a full explanation of the reason will be given towards the end of the saga, they are chosen to represent the different times and challenges I faced during my diagnosis, treatment and beyond. However, I'm sure many will guess my rationale behind this choice before the final chapter.

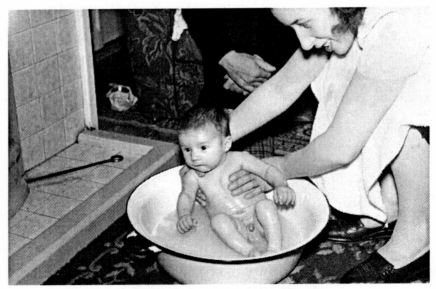

Who was to know what lay ahead?

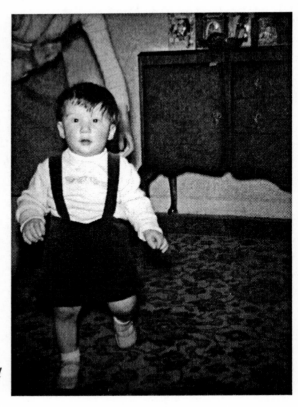

*That innocence would
soon be lost*

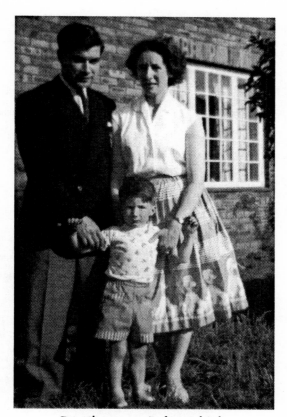

Proud parents, Ruby and John

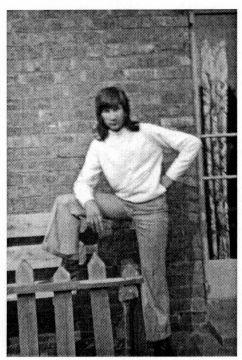

Looking in the future

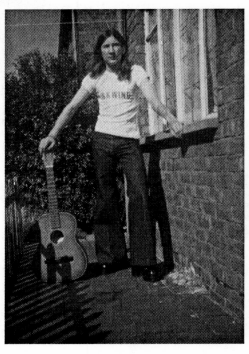

Ready to rock

Chapter Two

Later in the evening, the lights went out and the crowd erupted as Hawkwind took to the stage and the hairs on the back of my neck stood to attention as the band welcomed everyone to the Sundown.

Night Of The Hawks

Before we get into the essence of the story, I think it is important to set the scene; to describe a few of my early encounters and therefore offering you the reader an illuminative insight into my character, how it was before the spectre of cancer consumed my adolescence and then moulded my perspective of life forever and into the person I have now become.

Sometime towards the end of August, 1973 Robbo and I, accompanied by my father, headed across to the other side of the River Tyne to Walker where interviews were being held for apprenticeships in a number of the local shipyards. Shipbuilding was the mainstay of employment in the area back in the seventies and had been since the early Victorian era. The North East was always recognised as the world capital of Shipbuilding, particularly the Tyne, having produced quality and famous ships for centuries, the first of the super tankers, the Esso Northumbria, naval vessels by the score, including HMS Ark Royal and Illustrious to name but a couple. Sadly today, that industry has almost all disappeared.

By my own admission and as so many teenagers have followed on to do, I completely wasted my school years; although later in life I would make up for this lack of drive and educational ambition. Subsequently, I left school with a meagre selection of useless qualifications hoping to follow in my father's footsteps into Plumbing in a local shipyard. Unfortunately, the clear truth was that with my poor exam achievements I was not likely to be offered an apprenticeship in the field of plumbing.

I went into the interview, which was a little like a cattle market, one in, one out, next please, until they filled all of the vacancies. I sat and had a brief five minute lecture on the merits of the company's generosity and then, as an alternative to plumbing, I was offered an apprenticeship as a welder. In many respects, I was quite bewildered as to why I could not be a Plumber despite the qualifications I had proudly presented. However, still none the wiser why plumbing was not an option and realising that I had to map out a career of some description and secure a financial future for myself I accepted the job. Well, it was better than nothing and the pay wasn't too bad either, that was definitely an important issue. Furthermore, my father had explained the necessity of taking up such as post and I respected his view and therefore, in a few moments the indentures were signed and I was on the first rung of the employment ladder, but what an ascent it would prove to be.

And so it was that I had secured my first position of employment and the prospect of life as a welder. The first twelve-month were spent in a training school at Walker starting in September 1973. Not very glamorous nor was it particularly exciting. However, as an aspiring adult I now had cash in my pocket (first pay packet of £9.97), and the ability to realize one of my very first dreams, seeing Hawkwind live whatever it took.

Late in 1973, Sounds Magazine advertised what for me was a very special event, the next Hawkwind tour, just what I had desperately been waiting for. But regrettably, on closer scrutiny of the itinerary there was no Newcastle concert which was a devastating blow, even though they were playing just about every other corner of the country, Newcastle wasn't part of this tour. Therefore, there was only one thing for it, if they were not to visit the North East, then I'd have to travel somewhere to see them. Subsequently, I decided to see them at the now famous Edmonton Sundown in Silver Street, London early in the New Year. So, when I returned from work that night I sat down, put pen to paper, sent off my postal order, and stamped addressed envelope for the most important ticket of my short life.

The ticket duly arrived a week and a half later and I quite vividly recall sitting gazing at the maroon coloured ticket before leaving for work at 7am that Thursday morning. The following weekend I booked a travel ticket and a couple of days off work and made the eight-hour journey to London by coach. Naturally, I hadn't been so sensible to arrange accommodation during my visit to London, but what the heck, I would sort something out when I got there? Setting out from South Shields the coach trip seemed an endless journey such was my excitement on January 26th 1974, but the coach eventually arrived in the Capital. Of course, having never been to London previously I had little idea as to which direction to head in a bid to find the arena.

Three hours later, after much searching and enquiring I managed to find the Sundown. I had time to spare and got myself something to eat before making my way into the auditorium just as the support band were coming on stage, this was incredible, what an atmosphere, was I about to see Hawkwind after waiting so long? The air was filled with the sweet smell of cannabis yet, my adrenaline was flowing and I was on an artificial high of natural endorphins and euphoria.

Later in the evening, the lights went down and the crowd erupted as Hawkwind took to the stage and the hairs on the back of my neck stood to attention as the band welcomed everyone to the Sundown. Without further explanation, Hawkwind exploded into their first number, 'Brain-box Pollution', it was unbelievable as they continued their set and played without a pause between songs, while behind the band, there was a huge screen upon to which animated images where projected and which rep-resented each of the songs being delivered to an admiring audience. As they played, an amazing light show lit up the whole front of the stage and enhanced the performance. What an experience, what a show, the concert was awesome, much more than even I had expected, in fact there were not enough adjectives in my vocabulary to explain the brilliance of the gig, I was gob smacked, speechless and impressed as never before. At the end of the performance the crowd exploded with mesmerised appreciation as the band left the stage, returning minutes later to deliver an explosive encore, their final number being 'Silver Machine'. That night was something else, something you cannot explain to people, something that lives with you for the rest of your life, something only a Hawkfan can appreciate. But all too soon the concert was over and reluctant to leave I resentfully made my way out of the arena and through the streets of Brixton still buzzing with excitement and delirium and I felt like the 'Master of the Universe'. My desire and adulation to see more of the band was simply insatiable. Now walking through the streets of London, people passing by probably thought I was crazy, smiling to myself one moment, then remembering the song list and singing away to myself the next. What a high, who the hell needed drugs when such a rush could be gained in this way?

Unfortunately, I was about to fall to earth very quickly from this artificial high, as my problems would start late that January night. During that amazing Hawkwind concert I had had the good fortune to meet lots and lots of people, a bunch of Scottish guys had, like myself, come down by coach for the concert, a journey they had made previously. They were a good bunch and full of joviality and extremely friendly, they had told me that as their coach, like mine, wasn't due to leave until the next morning, then they had planned to allow themselves to be locked into Euston Station so that they could sleep there. This idea didn't fill me with much inspiration, although I was tempted and in hindsight I should have allowed my temptation to rule as I then made my way back to Victoria Coach Station. I had been told that at Victoria Coach Station, provided you had a valid ticket of travel you could sleep on one of the overnight-parked buses. Therefore, I headed back to Victoria, fingers crossed that this was indeed the situation.

I arrived at the Coach Station well after midnight; there were only a handful of coach's strewn indiscrimately in the now desolate station. It was true, one coach was allocated to those individuals using the transport the following day and I decided that this was obviously the warmest place I would find to sleep. I climbed aboard and secured one of the many empty seats. I had only been seated for around thirty minutes and I guess there were probably only half a dozen other people on the coach at this time with the same intent as I, or so I thought. Legs tucked up and covered with my afghan coat I felt fairly comfortable, that was until two adults and a young girl got onto the coach. Wrongly, I assumed that all three were together, unfortunately, I could not have been more off target. The lady and her daughter sat behind me and the man sat next to me despite all of the other empty seats available. However, in my naivety I didn't question this, thinking that all three were together. Moments later and a hand brushed against my knee. In my continued naivety I thought that this was a straightforward accident and I pushed away his arm. Sadly I was very wrong and this time his hand had a firm grip on my left leg. Realising with alarm what was happening I immediately jumped to my feet and forced my way passed this pervert and headed off the bus. The man remained firmly implanted in his seat as I took one final backwards glance.

Now shaking and frightened, I walked briskly out of Victoria Coach Station and wondered what to do on this extremely cold winter night. Dressed only in jeans, a t-shirt and an afghan coat, my hands felt numb from the bitterly cold January wind. Thankfully, I discovered the Salvation Army soup kitchen and made the best of what could have been a disturbing event. Even so, the predicament did not detract from my enjoyment of finally seeing Hawkwind live and early the following day I jumped on the bus to head back to the North East of England where I could not wait to tell Robbo and my other friends of the brilliance of the performance and of course the numbers they had played.

Today, I can laugh at that dangerous situation which might have had different consequences had the coach been completely empty. Naturally, it does quite clearly emphasize what a dangerous society we live in. Significantly, returning on the coach the following day, I remembered that one of the Scottish lads had a tattoo on his upper arm, it was a copy of a figure from Hawkwind's Space Ritual album and I had convinced myself that soon I would get the same tattoo done, this would demonstrate my commitment to the band.

Of course, having now experienced at first hand the band live, then this was never going to be enough of this visually stunning and amazing psychedelic band. Hawkwind offered something no other band could deliver. A unique blend of music, light shows (way ahead of their time and copied by many, but never equalled) and let's not forget an exotic dancer. No, for me, travelling around to see Hawkwind would almost become a full time career; in fact, I always had aspirations to join the band as one of the road crew. Sadly, that was never to be, perhaps if illness had not intervened that dream might have come to fruition, who knows? Instead, I had to make do with seeing the band play at many venues around this great country of ours. It also allowed me to make friends with other like-minded individuals.

Back at home and acknowledging that the Hawkwind tour was into full swing I browsed the tour itinerary pasted on my bedroom wall and I noticed they were to play Leeds University in mid February. A sudden inspiration, 'why don't I make the relatively short trip to Leeds to see that performance too'. As they were not playing Newcastle, It was the least I could do, and so I did, life was good.

Not long after the return from Leeds, Robbo had approached me to ask if I would be interested in going on a boating holiday to the Norfolk Broads. As I had money in my pocket and was still on a high from the Hawkwind gig, I gave it little thought and said yes. Although I had already travelled far and wide to see Hawkwind, this was my first expedition away from home.

And so, we set off to travel down to East Anglia by train and then on to collect the boat. The week away was one of freedom laughter and plenty rock music as almost every bar we attended had a band playing, or so it seemed. During that week and rather stupidly, Peter, one of the four guys who was on the trip asked Robbo to trim his hair before going out. Well, if you really knew Robbo, you would never have asked him to do that. Struggling to keep his face straight, Robbo took one look at me and of course I urged him on and then, silence, Peter sat there in total innocence, and then the unmistakable sound of the scissors could be heard to echo throughout the boat. Robbo had removed the largest chunk of Peter's hair, immediately reeling back in hysterical laughter to review his own artistry. Naturally, the rest of us looked at the now scalped area of Peter's head and did likewise. As you would expect, Peter did not see the funny side of things and started verbally insulting Robbo, this made things even funnier and the tears of laughter rolled down our cheeks. That was just one of the milder escapades of a great holiday.

Back at work and experience of working life in the training school revealed many new dimensions of social activity. A number of the other apprentices had girlfriends and amazed me with some of their tales and escapades. It just proved to demonstrate my innocence and naivety and that really, I had lots to learn about girls but also life generally.

Girls were never high on my agenda at that particular time and liaisons tended to be casual. Like most young lads I had a number of girlfriends but none proved serious. One girl, Michelle, really wanted much more than I was prepared to offer. Michelle was a pretty, quiet girl but her attentions became somewhat obsessive at times, calling me each night on the phone and regularly knocking at the door unannounced. On a number of occasions, especially if I were in the house alone, there would be a knock on the door, and if I noticed that it was Michelle, usually accompanied by one of her friends, then I would ignore the door and hide behind the sofa in case they peeped through the window, funny the crazy things you do. As nice as Michelle was, she was not the kind of girl I could introduce to my friends; her taste in music was Donny Osmond. Don't get me wrong, everyone is entitled to his or her own taste in music, it was just that I did not want to be associated with it. In my view, girls where not as important as my music.

Another girl was Lauren, the Mayors daughter and I immediately fell in love with her the first time I met her. I was astounded when I asked her out and she said yes. However, she broke my heart when she ended the relationship some six weeks later. You see, she was quite experienced, if you understand my meaning, experienced with the male fraternity, far more experienced than I was with the female gender and I think she was expecting me to be a little more forward and adventurous than I was. You certainly learn the hard way with girls.

My youthful looks would at times prove a hindrance. Seldom, if at all could I walk into a bar and get served and most often there would be a denial of access. Therefore, it was a matter of slipping into the corner and passing my cash to someone else to get the beers. The very first time I recall going to a bar, it was the Albermarle in 1973. I sneaked into the corner of the room and handed over my fifty pence to one of the lads. This was enough for four pints of Exhibition at 12 ½ pence per pint, good strong, northern beer. At last, I felt like a man, but also one of the crowd, but at the end of the night I was so drunk that I could barely walk and was guided by the lads into a taxi and sent on my way. Despite my drunken stupor I clearly recall stumbling into the front door at home, being aware that mam and dad where watching TV in the front room, therefore, I had no intention of going in there, they'll know immediately and boy would I have been for the high jump, I mumbled something about going straight to bed and fell on top off the bed and had the horrendous experience of the bed spinning before I dropped off to sleep, only to awaken the following morning with the hangover from hell. My first thought was, never again, not until the next time of course. Though they never said anything, I'm sure my parents new that I was drunk, parents just do. It's quite amazing how one can recall such events with such clarity, despite being well and truly inebriated.

Life in a shipyard brought many more friends and many more adventures. A typical teenager, dabbling in all that teenagers do, including my first experience of cannabis and LSD (acid), after all, it was the acid drenched seventies. However, before the shock horror and gasps of despair, please let me explain further, I was never into the drug scene heavily but in an honest account of the influential changes I have experienced it did play a small part and I do not intend to hide or falsify any aspect of what is written here.

Friday night, downstairs in the Ship and Royal was not only the place the local rockers met, myself included, it was the venue where a variety of drugs were exchanged for cash. Equally, I will not try and justify or argue the case of drug taking. For me and the circle of friends I associated with, Cannabis was smoked on a more than regular occurrence while personally, I only took LSD on a handful of occasions and probably only because of the as yet, unknown intervention of illness. As a great believer in fate, I would argue that things happen for a reason and had it not been for the intervention of cancer, what direction my life may have taken we will never know?

As a young man I admit to being rather immature and I think this was almost certainly a legacy of a wasted schooling, although I would make up for this later on in life. I do however, as I will more than likely reiterate time and time again, believe that fate governs our lives. When we are born I believe we are dealt a hand of cards and we have no option other than to play that hand of cards in the game that is life. Now that's putting things simply, I do believe that you cannot change your own fate, call it destiny if you like and yes, of course you can tempt fate by your own actions, but life is mapped out for us. It's a huge and naturally contentious issue, which importantly is my opinion. I certainly do not believe in forcing my opinion on anyone else in the same way I do not expect others to force their opinions, religious or otherwise onto me. Let's just accept each other for what we are and respect that as individuals we can make our own decisions. So I believe my fate was mapped out for me and being a scholar in those early days was not part of it.

Friends at work had similar tastes in rock music as myself and subsequently invited me to join them at their local pub. Evenings at the Marsden Inn would become an important social event on most nights of the week; I now had a group of friends that I could readily identify with. Not only did they enjoy my kind of music, but also we would take in regular live bands at a variety of venues around the region. Saturday night was rock discos at the Commando in South Shields market place, an upstairs room in a dishevelled pub, the sweet smell of hashish filling the air; this offered an important social event. A number of guys who attended the Commando were indeed, into stronger drugs such as Cocaine, significantly however, despite being an impressionable and immature teenager, I was consciously aware that that was not for me and I can guarantee that I was never ever tempted to try the harder substances. Despite being embraced into their fold for almost a year I would subsequently loose contact with my new found fraternity due to my imminent hospitalisation. Now, that is not to say that I didn't have any other friends, of course I did, it was just that they had different priorities than I did. Most importantly, they did not share my passion for rock music.

Some of the guys I'd made friends with and particularly a group from Whiteleas had some musical talent, in fact, a dam site more than I did. They had decided to form a band and had invited me to be the roadie and arrange the PA system and quite naturally, I jumped at the chance. After some months of impromptu rehearsals, an agent had arranged their first gig, a local workingman's club, but hey, this could be the first tentative step to rock stardom and I was part of it. Life was moving in a direction that gave me great pleasure, sadly however, there was something lurking just around the corner which would soon put a stop to my current enjoyment and which would take my life in a different direction.

The band felt as prepared as they could be and so we hastily made our way down the A19 in a beaten up old transit van which had seen better days, however, we had managed to persuade its owner of our desperate plight and he agreed to transport us to this most important event, hopefully the first of many gigs. It was at Shiney Row Club and on the night, a Saturday to be precise, everyone was on a high as we set up the stage and sound checked ready for the show at about 8.00pm. Naturally, being their debut the lads were nervous and subsequently required a little Dutch courage by the way of a few pints.

Before we new it, it was that time, the compere came on stage, stood to attention by his microphone and said, *"Please give a huge Penshaw welcome for Shelter"*. Rapturous applause came from the unsuspecting audience who sat back in eager anticipation. Of course, the agent who had booked the gig had informed the band that this was a 'rock night', which, as it turned out could not have been further from the truth. Onto the stage the lads marched as if gladiators being welcomed into the Roman Coliseum, quickly arming themselves with the appropriate musical instruments and then the guitar riffs blasted the introduction to 'Johnny 'B' Goode'. The lead singer jumped around the stage like a contorted epileptic, writhing and twisting before the first words came from his youthful throat. At the end of this number the singer was puffing and panting and I was doubtful whether or not he had the stamina for the rest of the show. Clearly, the muffled grunts and groans along with a muted applause told an entirely different story, this was no 'rock night!' more like 'Darby and Joan.' Still, in the good old show business fashion, the show must go on, unfortunately, the second number, an Allmans Brothers Band selection proved just as unpopular as the opening number and the compere was immediately onto the stage to put an end to the boy's performance and the noise that they had proudly presented. I cannot remember his exact words, which in any language meant 'get off'.

Of course, such was their embarrassment that they refused to go back on stage to clear away the equipment; instead that privilege was bestowed upon me and the other roadie. That was some experience clearing the stage to the ogling eyes of two hundred beer-swilling punters. One of the lads, Ralph, was so embarrassed that instead of leaving the building by the way we had entered; he decided to climb from the dressing room window and into the awaiting transit van. Meeting up with Ralph some thirty years later and he would profess to still being mentally scarred from the experience. But, on the way home we had a good old laugh about the entire proceedings and looked forward to the next gig, although at that time I did not know that that would be my first and last gig with the boys, but not by choice.

Despite my desire and urge for the rock lifestyle, I did have a good variety of friends, some of whom had little interest in rock music. There were occasions when I would still feel the need to go out with these other guys too. I think I was very lucky to have such a wide diversity of friends. On one occasion, Colin had suggested that as part of the celebration for Keith's bachelor stag night, then we should do something original, something that would turn the heads of others, something very different. Therefore, his suggestion was that we should go on a pub-crawl in fancy dress. Back in 1975 this was quite a novel idea and so we agreed, but fancy dress with a difference. Keith dressed as the Pope and the rest of us wore Nun's outfits. The night was a huge success and good fun, in fact, on the following Monday, the local tabloid, the Shields Gazette carried a story, '*Dancing Nuns and Vicars Hoax*', followed by the story that had captured the imagination of the revellers in South Shields.

There were certainly many escapades in the shipyards too and it was amazing that ships actually got built. One lad who was in the same year apprenticeship as Robbo and I was a guy called Plank; I'll let you decide why, as he was not the brightest bulb in the box and, on one occasion he fell asleep during an afternoon break so we welded the steel caps of his boots to the deck of the ship and left him to awaken in surprise. Another time a lad called Irish, a burner by trade was doing some work on the ships shell. He was supposed to be burning something off the inside of the shell; unfortunately he burned all the way through the wrong area of the shell causing water to seep in to where he was working. He was not popular when the foreman discovered his mistake, and that's putting it mildly.

Davey was a real nice guy, still is; his mistake was to set light to one of the other apprentice's newspaper as it lay beside him during an official break. Unfortunately, as the tabloid ignited it also caught the bottom of this other guy's boiler suit and his trousers were on fire. Although we saw the funny side of things, as did the victim, it could have been a very dangerous accident. Sadly for Davey the entire episode had been witnessed by one of the foremen and despite the support of the lad whose trousers had caught fire, Davey was sacked within the hour.

A 17-year-old lad enjoying life to the full. If this was what life was all about, having fun and following that amazing and progressive band, Hawkwind from tour to tour, then life was sweet. My goal at that moment in time was to get backstage and meet the band during their next tour, that was going to be a difficult feat, and so it would prove! The band had recently released their new album, 'Hall of the Mountain Grill' and one particularly track was very special, packed with emotion and incorporating haunting keyboards, 'Wind of Change', paradoxically, that's exactly what I was about to experience.

A couple of weeks later and it was time to purchase a ticket for the forthcoming Hawkwind tour; they had already completed a successful tour of America earlier in the year and now they were on the road again in the United Kingdom. This time I'd get to see them at Newcastle City Hall, as I would year in and year out. Sure enough, 12th December would prove a fantastic gig, if anything; they were much improved to earlier in the year, despite they're almost constant touring. Two days later and I travelled to Manchester to witness the band at the Palace and at that moment, life could not have been any better. Yes, life was cool, what more could a young man want from his existence? Had I not needed the commitment of work to finance my following of Hawkwind, then I would have simply made sure that I attended each show in each city of each tour.

Importantly, I had not forgotten about the tattoo that one of the Scottish guys I had met in London had on his arm, so I decided to take the specific Hawkwind album cover to a local tattooist and get the same done. Unfortunately, the tattooist said that the design I wanted would be quite difficult and he couldn't do it, of course I should have realised there and then that this guy was not reputable. But, as I had plucked up the courage to get the tattoo done in the first place I simply chose another design, a pirate's head. Yes, I am well aware of the stupidity of choice but I'd also had Dutch courage, alcohol. Days later and the tattoo was infected, my parents went crazy, but what was done was done and unfortunately, these things do not come off.

Into the new year and I decided to make the journey down to Dunstable as Hawkwind had once again decided to tour America later that year and it may be a while before I would get to see them again, how right that thought would prove to be, but not for the reasons I thought. Therefore in innocence, on the 13th April 1975 I did exactly that, travelled to Dunstable and the Queensway Hall. Sadly, despite a long and exhausting journey, the performance on this occasion was not the power packed space rock that I was becoming accustomed too, a somewhat indifference performance, or was it me? During the show I was unable to maintain a steady degree of concentration and my enthusiasm was waning, not for the band, far from it, it was more my physical well-being which seemed to be draining from my body, but what was causing my exhaustion? I had absolutely no inclination. But even so, I felt that my long trek south had not been in vain, I still had aspirations to join the band in some shape or form and understood that not every performance would be great.

Back at work and still exuberant from the gig I was slowly but surely beginning to realise that fatigue was consuming me physically, for a number of days now I had been feeling decidedly weak, even during my trip to Dunstable I hadn't felt wonderfully well and in hindsight, it was the euphoria of the concert and seeing the band live that had masked the overwhelming fatigue. The couple of weeks before my trip I had been struggling to motivate myself to go out after work and actually, most nights after work, I'd come home, eat with the family and then fall asleep in front of the fire. However, such was my enthusiasm to share my experiences of the concert that I did return to work following the Dunstable gig.

It was becoming increasingly more difficult to motivate myself to do anything at all and it seems that all I ever did was sleep, sleep and sleep. In addition, I had lost a significant amount of weight and although out of nothing other than ignorance I had no concern about this while at that moment in time I weighed a little over seven stones. Other symptoms included severe night sweats, night sweats that were so profuse that the entire bedding had to be changed. I had an intractable cough, which would eventually (once I was admitted to hospital) require methadone to settle it. In addition, I also developed breasts, (medically known as gynaemacostia), admittedly only small ones but again out of ignorance I thought nothing of it, furthermore, I had a yellow tinge (jaundice) to my skin. Significantly, I had already made a number of visits to my family doctor but he was about as much use as a chocolate fireguard, insisting that I was depressed and prescribing anti-depressants, Valium to be exact.

Following each meal and with increasing ferocity I would vomit, while most of the time I felt nauseated, but why? The doctor had no answers other than depression. An almost constant lethargy accompanied each moment of every day and sometimes I felt dizzy and disorientated. Strangely, I complained of having weak legs, a sort of tingling in the knees, although this did not affect my mobility.

I could not begin to describe the tiredness that enveloped my every movement. Even at rest I was completely exhausted and I accrued many sick days, but regardless, I made every effort to get into work. The Ship-yards were no different to any other industry; some people in positions of authority (foremen) took the role so seriously that it became an all-consuming pastime. In fact, so consuming that they treated all others with complete disdain, these dictatorial leaders gave the majority of foremen a bad and undeserved reputation. Of course for some of the foremen (heads of departments) then the position would lend itself ideally to justifiable ungentlemanly and offensive behaviour. However, many others in these apparently respected positions would play fairly with the workforce provided you completed your allotted work, which I suppose is understandable. For me however, life remained a joke and as an admittedly immature young man now just turned eighteen years of age, the main function of life was fun and being for the enjoyment of music, specifically Hawkwind.

Chapter Three

A diagnosis of cancer brings with it a change to every aspect, without exception of your life. Your thoughts divert off at tangents during the most inopportune moments and serve up a constant reminder that cancer is a life threatening disease. A convergence of negative and positive emotions, causing regular emissions of confusion and bewilderment.

Damage Of Life

May 1975 was a period of time that would forever change my life, the months and years that would shape my future, a time and experience that would mould my future philosophy and also my personal beliefs. The experience I was about to undertake would change my approach to each and every day and my life would forever be different than it otherwise would have been. This was my fate and it was to make such radical alterations to my own mind set that although I didn't know it at that time, I would eventually be eternally grateful and positively reflective of the journey I was about to embark upon.

Generally, I was quite happy despite the unexplainable lethargy that dominated my every breath. The current situation had now been going on for some six weeks; the family doctor appeared to be none the wiser as to the origins of my current symptoms and was unconcerned. I thought that if my family doctor was not concerned then surely I shouldn't be either and it would correct itself soon! I was enjoying a good social life; Hawkwind had yet another new album out called 'Warrior on the edge of time' and proved a real masterpiece, still a great favourite of mine today.

On one occasion at work, I was allocated a job in the cofferdams. These are the structures within the bowels of the ship, similar to the honeycombs of a beehive. The job would entail me physically dragging the welding cable down through the seemingly hundreds of manholes and into the double-bottoms. Naturally, there was no lighting down there and it was up to the individual to take a lamp with him so that the specific area could be identified. Trust me when I say, these cofferdams were well named; they were frightening places, black and deadly silent. Eventually reaching my allocated job and now, being completely exhausted I felt entirely washed out, so, I decided to sit and have a short rest before starting the welding job expected of me. It was now around 11.00 in the morning and not surprisingly, as you would expect, such was my fatigue, I fell sound asleep.

Some three hours later and I was awoken by one hell of a bang, the Foreman had found me asleep. Apparently, the siren had gone for lunch, everyone went to lunch and then returned. That was, everyone but me and of course this had not gone unnoticed. Jimmy the carthorse (certainly not a term of endearment, but most of the foremen had nicknames allocated by the workforce) was my foreman and he had come looking to see what kind of progress had been made with the job, particularly as far as he was concerned I had gone AWOL. He was not a happy chap when he had made his way down to were I was supposed to be working and found me sleeping like a baby. Fortunately for me Jimmy wasn't a bad foreman, there were many much worse. In fact, many others would have sacked me on the spot. What followed was the fiercest verbal lambasting I would ever receive. Still, it could have been much worse, in the situation, I could have easily been fired and not knowing how unwell I was, I knew that I had gotten off quite lightly.

The following day to my verbal rollicking I simply could not get out of bed as my weakness was getting steadily worse following another drenching night of sweats. I sincerely did try to motivate myself to get into work, knowing that after the previous day's rollicking, if I did not turn in, I could have lost my job. These sweats I mentioned were a specific symptom and caused such a degree of soaking that the bed sheeting needed to be completed changed as it was if someone had thrown a bucket of water over them.

Mum was working at the Scarlet Coat, a local and well respected restaurant, and knew I was too unwell to go to work and instead of trailing down to the doctors in person, she insisted that I rang them and insisted on a home visit. I agreed with her and later that morning the doctor arrived and immediately decided to have me admitted to the local hospital. He had suggested that my problem was appendicitis and that it probably required an operation, quite a change from his original diagnosis of depression, and yet, he was still way off target with his new diagnosis. He then insisted on calling an ambulance and a blue light flashed me to the Ingham Infirmary.

The first investigation was a simple blood test, although this would prove to be the first of many. Hours later and a blood transfusion was being arranged for me as it had been discovered that I was anaemic, a typical presentation of many haematological malignancies (blood cancers). Eventually, the doctor came along and placed a needle into the back of my hand without any explanation of the intended intervention, soon afterwards, the nurse turned up at my bedside holding the red bag of fluid, so much for consent then, so much for being informed. That same night a number of friends came in to see me and attempted to make fun of the situation but such was my weakness and lethargy that I could not be bothered with their joviality and found little fun in their antics, no matter how well intentioned. Still, it was nice that they had made the effort. Well, for the moment anyway!

Blood test followed blood test, followed by X ray, then onto the poking and prodding under my arms, squeezing my neck, then a hand on my stomach, the stethoscope on my chest and then on my back. Physical examination became a daily routine for a variety of doctors and of course, more blood tests. Despite the almost constant investigations in those early days, I remember that they were indeed, long, lonely days. On occasions, I thought that my body was no longer mine; such was the intensity of the constant intervention, the prodding and poking, and the constant barrage of the same questions, were they trying to catch me out in some way?

I remember vividly laying in a cubicle in the Ingham Infirmary with my radio playing and of course, it did not matter which radio station was chosen, there would be no Hawkwind to be found. Instead, I had to make do with radio one and other such commercialism; still it broke the monotony of those long tiresome days in what felt like solitary confinement. As if it were yesterday, I clearly recall the record, 'Loving You' by

Minnie Rippiton being aired. That record seemed to be on every ten minutes and it drove me to despair. Even today, if it's played on the radio it upsets me, as there is a direct association with those dark and dismal days. What others might consider to be a triviality, in that situation, feeling so desperately ill, then the disc jockey was playing this bloody record just to annoy me. Despite the uncertainty of any diagnosis at that time, the days were long and arduous, lonely and perplexing, uncomfortable and sad, was I becoming paranoid?

Where the hell was fate taking me? My exuberance was replaced by despondency, as I lay trapped in this hospital cubicle, the marching sound of mystery footsteps passing by without a word being spoken. Through the window of my internment a large expanse of lush green lawn was occupied by a family of blackbirds, searching the soil for worms and at the same time unconcerned at my personal plight, and beyond them I could see the silent movement of traffic heading out of the town. All alone, my mind was unequivocally confused and frightened; unsure as to what was happening, unaware as to why I was feeling so terrible.

Between investigations and when time allowed, some of the nursing staff would make any excuse to drop into my cubicle and chat. As most of them were quite young it was a welcome change to the mundane routine of my own company during those long painful and generally unhappy days. My despair was exacerbated by the fear of all these different investigations that I was enduring, what did they mean, what were they looking for?

The night sweats had not, and would not abate until treatment was initiated and continued almost nightly. Of course, the nursing staff were aware that this was a symptom of my condition, but as a naive and immature eighteen year old, I was terrified that the nursing staff would think that I had wet the bed due to incontinence. Silly really, but it's amazing what goes through ones mind at such a difficult time.

My diagnosis was one of four options, although the strongest suspicion was a malignancy, they were considering whether this was Tuberculosis, Infective Mononucleosis (Glandular Fever), Sarcoidosis or Hodgkin's Lymphoma. None of their suspicions however where relayed to me, perhaps they were waiting for a definitive diagnosis before they disclosed their findings? Then again, perhaps not.

It seemed that there was an almost constant tirade of investigations and I was perplexed as the nature of their search as explanations to me were not readily forthcoming. I suppose in many respects that one could argue that I should have asked, but in all honesty, I was prepared to let them get on with it in the hope that once a conclusion had been reached I would be the first to know, but from my perspective, this was the wrong assumption. In addition, I was not a very confident young man and therefore, I was content to let them get on with their search.

Then there was the daily ritual of at least one doctor coming to see me with the very same questions that had been asked the day before and once a week there would be an entourage of white coats dutifully following the consultant, all wanting to push here and squeeze there, listen to my chest and then looking perplexed. Meanwhile, one of the swellings (lymph nodes) was surgically removed from my neck; the lump was the size of a walnut and was excised under local anaesthetic and this proved a painless operation, but not all other procedures would prove so innocent or indeed painless. The lump was then sent for microscopic examination.

On Tuesday, my bowels would be put through their paces in the search for a conclusion to my illness. The unpleasant and nauseating 'Barium Swallow' was a disgusting white concoction that tasted of, well, nothing I'd tasted before and it certainly was not savoury I can assure you. The barium is impermeable to X Rays and therefore, it is used to highlight abnormalities in either the stomach or the bowel after a series of X Rays have been being taken. On Wednesday, my bowels were taken to the next level of investigation when once again the radiology department would seek new ways to explore the inner depths of my colon. Into the X Ray room I was taken, unknowing what to expect from this next exploration. Laying on my side the radiographer tells me of her intention, a plastic tube is placed into my backside and barium is pumped in there as if they were seeking to insulate my innards. As I am sure you can imagine, not very comfortable and I can certainly confirm that it was not an enjoyable experience, but it didn't stop there. No sooner did the barium flow into my bowels like cavity wall insulation than the table I was lying on started to twist and turn like a fairground attraction. Apparently, this spinning and turning would enable a new series of films to see my bowel at different angles.

The next day, I was taken across to the newly built diagnostic centre located at South Tyneside General Hospital for what was supposed to be one of the most important investigations which would rule out one diagnosis, but help to confirm another diagnosis. I was taken into a small cubicle were I was met by the Consultant Oncologist (of course, I didn't have a clue what this fancy title meant) who explained the procedure. I am told, it's a bone marrow investigation, well, that didn't sound too bad, or was the Consultant just a good salesman? The Consultant went on to ask if I had any objections over the junior doctor doing the procedure. To me, a doctor was a doctor, what difference could it make? Wrong! The junior doctor had no problem placing the local anaesthetic into the skin around my sternum (breastbone) where the biopsy was to be taken from. However, he struggled and struggled and then struggled some more to get any kind of leverage onto the special biopsy needle he was using and which was supposed to extract a sample of the bone marrow from my delicate skeleton. His struggle was such that he actually climbed onto the investigation couch with me to force more pressure on the needle. Yes, local anaesthetic had been used but, either he hadn't put enough of the dammed stuff in there or he had been a butcher in a previous life, alternatively, I was just a wimp. Seriously however, I was now struggling to tolerate the investigation and I think the Consultant realised this and he took over the job and got the required sample in a few minutes. Thank God that was over; I felt my chest was about to collapse like wet tissue paper. Back to the Ingham Infirmary for a much needed rest and a large helping of painkillers.

A couple of days later and it was at that juncture in time that my parents were taken to one side and told the news that all parents fear. My diagnosis was a malignancy, although definitive histology was still awaited, it appeared to be a cancer called Hodgkin's disease and the outcome (prognosis) was far from favourable, less than a 50% chance of surviving such was the extent of the disease, and that really depended upon how I responded to the treatment, failing to respond to the treatment would diminish the long term chances of survival even further.

Lymphoid tissue malignancies are grouped into one of two diseases, those being Hodgkin's Lymphoma, previously termed Hodgkin's Disease and all other lymphomas referred to as Non Hodgkin's Lymphomas. These are uncommon cancers of the lymphatic system and are of unknown cause, while Hodgkin's lymphoma is most common among fifteen to thirty year olds with a higher incidence amongst males. Thomas Hodgkin first described the disease way back in 1832.

Mam and dad were told by the Consultant that he would have liked to have seen me much earlier, and he was rather confused and angered as to why I had been put on Valium and not referred to the hospital! But regardless of the Consultants bewilderment to the delay and the strange prescription of Valium by the family doctor, what absolutely amazed me was the fact that back then (1975), the Consultant encouraged my mum and dad not to tell me of the diagnosis, *"we'd rather John didn't know his diagnosis"*, something that my mum and dad didn't need a lot of encouragement to undertake. To me this was out of order, thankfully it wouldn't happen today, or shouldn't happen today. Now don't get me wrong, I understand exactly why my mum and dad were happy to go along with this, there is no worse sensation in the world than being told your child has cancer, but that doesn't mean I agree with the sentiment. In fact, even today, there is often a healthy debate over the merits of this approach and so it turned out that I was not told of my diagnosis, denied the opportunity to be involved in the decision making process, to have at least some small degree of control as to what was and would be happening to me, was that too much to ask for? That decision by proxy still causes me great concern even today. Obviously, neither the Consultant or my parents had heard of the veracity principle, which highlights the ethical obligation to tell the truth, nor the underlying principle of patient collaboration which clearly regards the patient as being capable of making suggestions and of being involved in the decision making process, the patient should have a voice!

After the diagnosis, my father visited his father to tell him of the devastating news and he responded by informing my dad that he had money in the bank and that if it was needed, it could be used to search out the best treatment that would afford me the best opportunity of getting well. My father did not take up this option and he and my mum placed their trust in the local hospital and its dedicated staff.

Having already decided to exclude me from my diagnosis, the greatest concern now for my parents, was the fact that there was another patient on the same ward as I was and they definitely did not want me anywhere near him, although unknown to them, that was too late. I was undergoing all of these investigations to conclusively determine the cause of my symptoms while Joe had already been diagnosed with Hodgkin's lymphoma some five years earlier and was currently very poorly, in fact he was terminally ill and sadly died during that admission. Only days prior to his death, another patient and I had sat with Joe and although I wasn't aware of either his diagnosis nor his terminal state, even to my untrained eye, I could clearly see he was not a well man. My mum in particular was especially concerned in case I discovered his underlying diagnosis and that I would then be upset over his condition if I inadvertently found out about my own diagnosis, the diagnosis that was currently being hidden from me. This kind of problem of course can always happen when you try and collude to deceive an individual, even though that deception is well intentioned.

Furthermore, mam and dad had decided not to inform my younger sister, Allyson about my diagnosis. Now, once again, you can debate the merits of this, but, as Allyson was only thirteen years old, I could clearly understand their rationale for this move. It would be almost three years later before she realized that the condition could have easily claimed my life. Interestingly, Allyson would later confirm that she herself was pleased that she was not told, claiming that she would have struggled to come to terms with it. However, she could equally see things from my perspective and how frustrated I was at being declined the information that I was entitled too in the first instance.

Strangely, it seemed that all of a sudden, very few of my friends came to visit me, even when I eventually got home, the boys where noticeable only by their absence. It transpired that my mum had bumped into my best friend, Robbo on the local bus and had told him that I had cancer.

Of course, it wasn't long before most of my friends were made aware of this stigmatising diagnosis and I later found out that the reason they didn't visit was their fear of the word cancer and not knowing what on earth they could talk to me about. Perhaps the look on their faces would give the game away and I would jump out of the bed when I realised I had the filthy disease of cancer. Still, I can see why they were so fearful and I certainly do not hold any grudges toward them. Until we are in those specific situations, we simply do not know how we are going to react; perhaps it's the inability to confront our own mortality.

One of the biggest dilemmas with a cancer diagnosis is the fact that many, although not all people, do not appear to look unwell. It is the ultimate hidden poison, a denizen from the unknown. And so it was that many of my friends would say that very thing. You do not look as though you have cancer, but what does a cancer patient actually look like? It is no respecter of creed, colour or social standing, everyone is at risk and deep down inside, the scourge of society takes its toll on a defenceless body and is indiscriminate with its choice.

Prior to starting any treatment I was transferred to Newcastle General Hospital for a couple of additional tests, which would determine specific issues relating to the condition. It was now that I was admitted to a specialist ward for cancer patients, yet as few had lost their hair and I guess out of ignorance and naivety I did not realise that this was the ward that **all** cancer patients attended. However, whilst in Newcastle General I overheard one of the doctors discussing my case with another and just by pure chance happened to hear the diagnosis of Hodgkin's disease. Now this actually meant nothing whatsoever to me and I didn't give it a second thought. By pure coincidence the following day I bought a newspaper, fate had decided to take a hand and intervened. One particular story in this tabloid would not only shock me, it caused me great heartache, and it erupted my emotions, while at the same time I felt an implosion in my mind following this unexpected discovery.

Flicking through the paper I came across a headline that said *"A Crossroads Star Tells His Sad Secret"*. The character and wheelchair bound Sandy, played by Richard Tonge in the soap opera 'Crossroads' "had been hiding a grim secret from millions of fans"; he was fighting his own battle against Hodgkin's disease. Now this interested me, as I suddenly realised that this was the same condition as the doctors had said I had. Frighteningly, the article went on to reveal that Hodgkin's disease was cancer! That can't be right? Why did no one tell me? My mind raced, my head was spinning with confusion, and I experienced a kaleidoscope of emotional turbulence. A whirlwind of changing feelings, nothing could have prepared me for such a shock, perhaps I had misheard! Perhaps they had been talking about someone else! Except, deep down, I knew they had been discussing me. **I had cancer!**

Without doubt, this was a roller coaster ride that I'd never ridden before and I wanted to get off quickly, one moment you're up, the next you're on the bottom and without any control of what was now controlling me, my breath shortened and my heart bumped so loudly that I'm sure the patients in the next ward would have heard it, I was fearful and panicking, what was happening to my senses? From the depths of despair, to an almost euphoric excitation and then a tearful inexplicable depression. Anger! How dare that GP say I was depressed, what an affront that my so-called friends stayed away just at the time when I needed them most. Frustration! How on earth can I cope with a life threatening illness? Suicidal! What the hell is the point of having treatment for what is a killer disease? Pissed off! How dare my parents treat me like a child and keep this information from me. Ashamed! Disgusted at getting this most ugly of conditions. Fearful! Would I be around to see the future? Doomed! As far as I was concerned, people don't recover from cancer. Determined! I had so much to live for and boy did I want to live. Grateful! At least it was me, not my younger sister. So many emotions happening at the same time and so few people to help me deal with them. Tearful! And yet I didn't know why. Focussed! I needed an inspiration and I had exactly that in Hawkwind. Sad! There were times, many many times when it was just impossible to control my emotions.

My mum was quite flabbergasted when she came into hospital to find that I knew about the diagnosis, my diagnosis. She had come to visit with my dad and a couple of relatives. I wanted answers and really didn't get any, besides that was not the time to argue. In addition, and paradoxically, I could understand why they did what they did, even so, that still didn't make it right. More importantly, I honestly didn't feel as if I had any fight in me, or what little I had, then I was going to need for the long arduous battle ahead.

Trying to change the subject and divert attention away from the collusion issue, mam blamed the tattoo that I had had done a few weeks earlier and which had become infected. Naturally, there was no evidence for this but I could understand her desire to find something to blame. What made matters worse for me was the fact that I hadn't even gotten the tattoo that I wanted in the first place. I wanted a Hawkwind tattoo and ended up with this ridiculous pirate's head.

A diagnosis of cancer brings with it a change to every aspect, without exception of your life. Your thoughts divert off at tangents during the most inopportune moments and serve up a constant reminder that cancer is a life threatening disease. A convergence of negative and positive emotions would cause regular emissions of confusion and bewilderment.

Before discharge from ward 38, at Newcastle, another blood transfusion was arranged as I was found to be anaemic again such was the aggressive nature of the cancer. On the day of discharge I was started on a course of steroids, Prednisolone 10mg three times daily and also a drug called Procarbazine, 50mg three times daily. The ultimate plan was chemotherapy, but with so many different drugs being available to the clinician, it was essential that the correct combination was selected. The medical fraternity still needed more information so that correct choice of drugs could be selected so that I had the greatest chance of beating this aggressive disease. Subsequently, the two drugs I had commenced would at least begin to exert some affect on the cancer. Additionally, once all of results were available and irrespective of which chemotherapy drugs I would be given, then the steroids and the Procarbazine would form part of that treatment.

Although not being aware of it yet, I would develop a very important relationship with ward 38 at Newcastle General Hospital, but that would be many years later. It would not only be instrumental in my illness, it would be significantly influential in my future career.

Two days later and I awoke to find my body covered in an unexplained rash which caused me to want to scratch and peel my skin from the bones. Mam contacted the hospital and I was readmitted to South Tyneside for investigation and although I was not feeling terribly well, I could not say I felt any worse than the previous night when I'd gone to bed. Despite this and an absence of other typical symptoms, the medical staff thought that this may well have been meningitis and I was therefore isolated and had the usual barrage of blood tests. Happily, this turned out not to be the case, it was a simple drug reaction to the Procarbazine and after stopping the drug it soon settled down after twenty-four hours and the appropriate treatment. Once again, I was on my way home.

Chapter Four

Then, although it sticks in the back of my throat I bravely ask the question that I'm dreading the answer to: 'Am I going to get better from this?'

Standing On The Edge

The proposed treatment for this condition was the dreaded chemotherapy which was due to start the following Thursday as an outpatient at South Tyneside Hospital. Everyone has heard of that chemotherapy
treatment, hair loss, lethargy, vomiting and eventually you die, that was my
perception anyhow and the days leading up to Thursday's appointment, my
mind was filled with thoughts of this terrible chemotherapy treatment that
I was supposed to receive. Despite being admittedly immature, I wasn't
completely stupid, I had seen television programmes about people with
cancer and had seen the torture and torment they went through with this
chemotherapy treatment and that terrified me. On Thursday, I attended
the outpatient department and almost immediately I was taken into a
cubicle, not just any cubicle though, it was the same cubicle where the bone
marrow investigation had been carried out only a couple of weeks earlier.

The Consultant came in and passed the usual pleasantries and, in hindsight, his distraction therapy was very good as I gave very little thought to
the tray of large injections that lay only inches away from me. He lifted the
needle that he intended to place in my forearm ready for the delivery of the
proposed drugs and before I know it he has access to my venous system.
It really is quite strange the things our minds allow us to remember and
forget, but it is with crystal clarity that I can still see that very first injection, almost in slow motion moving towards my arm, the rapid beat of
my heart a clear indication that my fear was rising, unsure as to what the

reaction to these drugs would be. Slowly he began to inject the destructive substance known as chemotherapy. The drugs went in quite uneventfully, rating a zero on the scale of excitement. My initial thought was that this chemotherapy was a bit of a breeze, not the terrible treatment I had been led to believe, no problem, not what I had imagined at all, was I being overtly optimistic? Irrespective, my main thought was, would it be able to stem the cancer? That was the million-dollar question and no one could give an answer to that.

I do believe that much of the fear and stigma relating to cancer treatments must be laid at the door of the media. How sad it is when they could have an educative effect on the public, but all too often they tend to sensationalise cancer and its necessary treatments. What a great shame when someone comes along and is given a cancer diagnosis and told they need to have chemotherapy, then feel psychologically destroyed having previously read in a tabloid or watched a television programme that portrayed the event so negatively. Naturally, I am not saying that cancer and its difficult treatment's are easy to get through or that it is not a serious issue, of course it is. I just feel very strongly that most, although not all of the media do not report cancer facts accurately. All too often there is a sense of melodrama because this sells newspapers or is good television. That cannot be right if it is distorted to the degree that it gives the incorrect perception to those undergoing or about to undertake treatment for a cancer diagnosis. The media have a responsibility to report matters precisely and without prejudice to its honesty that potentially can cause psychological hurt to others if it is not!

The drug regimen I was to receive was called 'MOPP', an acronym of the drugs to be utilised, Mustine (Nitrogen Mustard) 8mg, Oncovin (Vincristine) 1.5mg Procarbazine (Natulan) 50mg and Prednisolone 40mg. The plan was to have six courses (cycles) of this treatment and each would be administered at three weekly intervals.

There had, in retrospect, been no informal or formal consent for this treatment to be given. Neither had there been any explanation of what I was to expect of the time after the chemotherapy had been administered. This is in my view, one of the most important reasons why such stigma is attached to cancer treatments, simple explanation of the potential side effects is vital and can allay so much fear from the patient's perspective. What's more, providing patient's with written information was unheard of back in the seventies and yet it is a vital component of empowering patients.

So my first chemotherapy treatment was now behind me and I planned to head off home. At the time, my granddad lived just over the road from the hospital and he obviously knew of my diagnosis and had told my dad that if I felt up to it I should call in after the inaugural treatment. I didn't really need a second asking as my grandad was in both the first and second world wars, in fact he was a prisoner of war during world war 1 and had some fantastic stories to tell, therefore, after my first treatment I called in to see him for thirty minutes or so. After this I headed home, only ten minutes away in a taxi. At home, mum had prepared one of her famous homemade mince pies. Of course, the steroids I was currently taking ensured my appetite was voracious and the pie was devoured in no time and I could not believe the negativity that went hand in hand with chemotherapy. Chemotherapy, this was pretty straightforward and not what I had expected, or did my optimistic anticipation come too soon? Of course it did!

No more than twenty minutes later and to say that I was sick is perhaps the biggest understatement so far. Projectile vomit from deep down within and I felt that my stomach had been turned inside out. In addition, it was not just a matter of being sick, emptying the contents of ones stomach and that was that, no, the retching continued for hours, which then stretched into days, many days. During the night the nausea was unbearable and the moment I got out of bed to visit the toilet, the very action of moving caused repetitive retching which by this time yielded nothing but bile and brash which lasted for almost a week. Unable to eat in fear of the sickness, my resolve was just about destroyed; I had never imagined anything like this and I could not believe that anyone could feel this way. The only anti-sickness medication way back then was a drug called Metoclopramide which was useless at controlling the side effects of treatment, and although this is still used today, it is either reserved for those drugs not expected to cause much in the way of sickness or in combination with other anti-sickness drugs.

Only two days after my first chemotherapy and I was back in hospital, but not because of the persistent nausea and vomiting, I awoke one morning to find that I had the biggest lips that cosmetic surgery could buy. What had happened was that I developed an allergic reaction to one of the cocktail of drugs I was taking and again, the Procarbazine was implicated. It seemed strange to me that the drug I had reacted too previously was given to me again? Significantly, the Procarbazine was a vital ingredient of the treatment regimen and therefore, they had decided to re-challenge my body with it. This treatment was so unforgiving, was there anything it could not do to your body systems? However, after ant-histamine treatment and just a few days later, those rubber lips had diminished.

The biggest problem with chemotherapy back in the seventies was that your body simply did not respond to commands, I was no longer in control of it. It was instructed by the chemotherapy and I was like a drug fuelled robot, an alien being with my actions controlled by the toxic drugs.

The treatment was repeated every twenty-one days, but there were only ten of those days that I felt reasonably well when I could put it to the back of my mind. Thankfully and without exception my friends began to come and visit. Once word got around that I was home, and others had visited without falling into the vast chasm of silence and the fear of saying the wrong thing, then others felt able to confront me, the friend with the big 'C'.

In fairness and without exception, my friends were supportive and indeed very protective. Later, in months to come when I would eventually feel strong enough to get out and socialise, the lads, almost without exception would demonstrate big brother protection. If I was pushed the wrong way, even innocently, then there was always someone there to ensure that it was accidental and I was safe. I very much appreciated this protection, feeling very fragile but also at times a little like royalty. Significantly, there were never any incidences of actual fights or other trouble, but I know that there was always a careful eye focussed on me.

Much to my own disgust and absolute sadness, I found handfuls of hair on my pillow one morning and without a second thought decided to get my hair cut. Well, it was pointless having long black locks that was certain to drop out as more and more of the dammed poison was pumped into my veins. I found this particularly hard to accept, as this long hair was an important part of my identity, my persona. Even my identity, as I saw it, was being eroded. At a later point in time, I would destroy just about every photograph of myself during that difficult time.

Naturally, I was feeling quite low at that moment in time and I required a sick note for work and unfortunately, had to visit the doctors. There was no way I was going to see that imbecile that had had the effrontery and guile to talk about something he knew nothing about, the man who stated that I was depressed. Instead, I asked to see the other doctor in the practice. However, I was just as taken aback when I went in to see her. She looked me in the eyes having signed my sick note and said, *"Have they told you your diagnosis"*? Before I had a chance to reply, she blurted out *"You have leukaemia"*. My, my, my, this was some medical practice, the doctors just make it up as they go along I'm sure. I informed her that this was not correct and made my way hastily to the door. At home I explained to my mum what had been said and she was so enraged that she rang the practice demanding to speak with the doctor. Luckily for the doctor she had gone out on house calls but this was probably just as well because I would not like to have been in the doctor's shoes if mum had gotten the chance to speak with her. One of the most important lessons my sister and I learned early in life was that you do not answer my mother back. Mum did speak with the receptionist and told her exactly what she thought of the doctor's lack of communication skills, so I am sure it would have gotten back to her.

Days before my next chemotherapy treatment was due again and I began to feel physically sick, knowing exactly what I was about to experience, sickness and vomiting, twisted bowels and an inability to eat food for days, well, not so much an inability to eat food, more of a fear to eat food as it was obvious what was going to happen. Apart from that, well it was a breeze, nothing to it really! If only that were true. I never knew this foreign substance deep within my veins could cause effects I'd never even dreamed about in my worse nightmare, a bloody storm of unforgiving proportions.

The day finally came when I was to attend the day unit at South Tyneside Hospital for the next chemotherapy treatment. I got there in plenty of time and had my bloods taken and made my way around to the waiting area and at first, I was saddened at what I saw, so many old folk. No, not the saddened sight of old folk, I thought of these old people having worked all of their lives and enjoyed what life had to offer only to be blighted by this terrible affliction that is cancer. Yet, here we all were without much control over this dreaded of diseases, irrespective of age, creed or colour. Such negative thoughts and I began to think of my own mortality and whether I would be around for the next Hawkwind tour, if I was, would I be well enough to sit through a concert without feeling sick.

In the background a voice shouted my name and it was my turn to see the Consultant for my treatment. I sluggishly dragged my feet into the consulting room to be faced by Dr. Sheppard who was a pleasant enough guy in hindsight; it was just that I didn't feel very much like being pleasant knowing what it was that I was there for. At the risk of sounding rude, although that is not my intention, he reminded me of Jerry Lewis in the starring role of the film the 'Nutty Professor' dressed in his long white coat, he had his glasses perched on the end of his nose and he peered over the top of them at me, a slight overbite he frowned as he stood along side me as I lay on the couch, his feet were clad in open toed sandals. Following a brief chat, he would twist his face up just as the 'Nutty Professor' did in the movie. Then following a physical examination, he tells me that my bloods are satisfactory, the lumps in my neck and axilla have started to go down and that the next treatment will be going ahead as planned.

Then, although it sticks in the back of my throat I bravely ask the question that I'm dreading the answer to: '*Am I going to get better from this?*' Now, I can't remember his exact words; come to think of it I can't remember any of his words, only the interpretation and I think looking back his answer was what is commonly referred to as spin, also called bullshit. What I do recall is that I was none the wiser following his response. But then perhaps I didn't want to know and I decided to allow fate to take its course. In my opinion, what I didn't know couldn't hurt me and therefore, I didn't pursue it any further.

Before I new it I had a steel needle in the back of my hand and ready for the toxic drugs to be pushed in. There were three drugs given into the needle, the first an anti-sickness injection, although I'm bewildered as to why it was called an anti-sickness injection because it was about as much use as my family doctor (and we know how good he was). The second seemed a huge injection which was called Mustine and was responsible for the nausea and vomiting and the third drug called Vincristine had the most weird taste sensation as it was being administered, not only could I taste it, I could also smell it. This was just unbelievable, and trust me when I say that it was not a pleasant taste, it was a foul metallic taste unlike anything I'd ever experienced. During subsequent injections I would have a large glass of orange to sip very slowly while the drug was being given and although it didn't take the taste away in its entirety it did help.

During the treatment my heart raced and I felt tearful. I suppose it was the anticipation, the fear of the unknown, but also the fear of the known, knowing that the violent sickness lay just around the corner and of course, something I believe is typical of most cancer patients, the uncertainty of what lay ahead in my future, did I have a future?

And so, on completion of the chemotherapy for the second time, I headed home feeling unsure about how and indeed, if I wanted to continue with this infernal treatment. At this particular moment in time however, I did not feel that I had any other option than to continue, at least for the time being. This is something that would plague me on and off for months until there was an inner conflict and self-confrontation. Additionally, I decided not to call into my grandad's as I didn't want to start feeling sick in his house, after all he was in his late seventies and that would have been unfair. Once at home I decided to eat only a light snack as this had been the trigger following my first treatment, the doctor had changed the anti-sickness medication this time so I was hopeful that I did not suffer as I did with my first treatment, fingers crossed.

Sadly, and within a couple of hours I knew that feeling, even though I'd only experienced it once previously, there was no mistaking. Following the predatory attack of the chemotherapy on my system, my stomach was preparing to erupt like an active volcano waiting to spontaneously spew its contents for the first time. Sure enough, a crescendo of nausea and then the sickness started and my stomach was soon aching as it had three weeks earlier. All I could do was to retire to the bedroom, close the curtains and play some Hawkwind and it probably sounds silly to most people, but not only could I identify with the band, having now seen them play live, but also the music allowed me a greater sense of escapism and I suppose most importantly, distraction. I lay on the bed confined by my chemical straightjacket with no escape.

Irrespective of your situation, everyone, I believe needs inspiration and motivation, but Hawkwind are far more than simple inspiration; they are, as many will testify, a way of life, to love them is to be part of them. In addition to the music, the experience is pure escapism, a romantic affair with creation and invention. In many respects, despite giving my fervent support to Captain Dave Brock and all who have aided and assisted his direction of the band over the years and I could never repay what I owe them following the support I have taken from the band over the years.

Therefore, I was naturally pleased to read that the band was planning a tour later in the year and this gave my deflated persona some much needed inspiration, more importantly, as part of the tour they were due to headline at the now famous Reading rock festival and it was my intention to be part of that experience, to soak up the atmosphere, a free spirit destined to be part of the Hawkwind experience and the thought of this new phenomena was a great driving force for me.

I was struggling to come to terms with this evil cancer and at times my mind was constantly buzzing, a fear of the savage attack of the chemotherapy, what was the point of adding to my woes by worrying, but that was easier said than done as I could quite simply not control the strange and fearsome thoughts lingering in my mind. Yet at other times I felt ashamed at the way I was feeling sorry for myself, in fact, there were times when I wanted to give myself a good kicking to try and pull myself together. I knew deep down, despite being an immature eighteen year old, that I had to stay focussed and positive. In addition, it was unfair to my very supportive family. Indeed, it was unfair to Hawkwind, I saw myself as the number one fan (still do) and I couldn't let them down.

Between treatments I had family and friends visit on a regular occasion but more often than not I simply could not be bothered with visitors, as I felt obligated to make conversation. Not only that, in particular, my friends were always talking about the nights out, what they had been up to and of course the sticky scrapes they'd get themselves into. I felt more depressed after their visits as I was becoming aware of what I was missing out on, the excitement and mischief of adolescence, including girlfriends. At other times this talk actually fuelled my motivation to try and beat this horrendous illness.

It was a lonely time when isolation played weird mind games with my psychological status. But importantly, I found this a time of personal reflection and self assessment, a time to take stock and to appreciate life itself. A time when I was thinking about things that I'd never considered previously. Acknowledging that life is made up of simple, but beautiful things and which we often do not appreciate. The myriad of glistening stars floating in the infinite darkness of space and equalled in number only by the grains of sand on South Shields beach. Appreciating the hypnotic beat of the unrelenting waves as they pound the unprotected shoreline without relent. Up above, the marshmallow clouds drifting effortlessly across the sky as a variety of birds soar on the invisible thermals beneath, the rhythmic echo of raindrops on the window as you lay in bed. Louis Armstrong was exactly right when he said, "and I think to myself, what a wonderful world."

After were born, the only certain fact in life is that one day we will die, the only variance for us is when that will be. Often, it is only after some life changing experience that we consciously reflect on life generally and appreciate its significance, it's sanctity, it's beauty and of course, it's uniqueness. Have you ever taken time to sit and admire the everyday world? The wind rustling through the ancient branches of an old oak tree. Then of course, there is nothing more impressive than the first snow flurry of winter, taking a handful of virgin snow and feeling each of your fingers tingle to numbness. What a fantastic world this is, yet we know so little about life itself! So many things to admire about being alive, so many things to fear, but ultimately, what is life all about? Sadly, no one has that answer. Confronting your own mortality has a strange way of raising many intriguing issues.

A cancer diagnosis also elicits the bereavement process, grief and feelings of loss are not just reserved for those individuals who have lost loved ones. Following a diagnosis of cancer one goes through a multitude of recognised emotions, Denial, (this can't be happening to me, it's a dream), Anger, (why me, I've never done anything to deserve this), Bargaining, (I will live my life respectably and go to church if only I'm ok), depression, (something I would become accustomed too), acceptance, (if this is my time then I have to deal with it). Of course many people go through these emotions in many different ways and not necessarily in this order either and many of the emotions are re visited too. But at this particular juncture in my life, I felt as though I matured very quickly, appreciating that life indeed, is a beautiful thing.

At times it was easy to be positive and to look forward to the future. However, at other times I felt weak for allowing seeds of doubt to invade my mind and promote negativity about my own future. I was consciously aware of my own body image and it wasn't very good, I knew the importance of gaining some weight to improve my seven stone stature. Weighing myself everyday became an obsession, yet the weight proved extremely difficult to put on as I continued to feel grotty, fatigued, nauseated and what's more food tasted lousy. Subsequently, the task of gaining weight would prove hard in the short term, it was a vicious circle, for that moment in time, a no win situation.

I thought of life as a whole host of small islands of happiness surrounded by a deep sea of shit. You get onto one island and enjoy the happiness it has to offer, but all to often the tide swamps the island and you once again are left in the sea of shit until you can drag yourself onto the next island, this epitomised my predicament.

When the time came to go back to hospital for further treatment my mind was twisted and full of fear and indignation and no matter how hard I tried I just could not escape the negative thoughts in the back of my mind. Entering the hospital and my body felt like a lonely, trembling leaf on the branch of a huge tree waiting for the autumnal breeze to take control of it. Concerned and anxious about the pending treatment I attended the blood room and had the requisite samples taken before heading round to the yellow waiting area at the hospital. That in itself compounded the anxiety and fear, as there was a compulsory wait for the blood results before a decision on whether treatment would go ahead.

Then, the nurse shouted my name and in I go, the bloods are within the normal ranges, which meant the chemotherapy could be given. However, just before the chemotherapy is given there is the inconvenience of the physical examination. As I was lying on the examination couch I knew that I was close to tears of anger and uncontrollable panic and even though it was still early days in my cancer journey I knew that feeling, the anguish, the doubt at my own resolve and I knew I was beginning to falter. The chemotherapy was brought into the room that had my frail body lying uncomfortably on the couch and the nurse provides me with a large glass of orange to take away that horrible metallic taste and uncanny smell, created so paradoxically by the Vincristine as it was administered.

No sooner had the Consultant began to push the cocktail of drugs into my system that my stomach began to gurgle and churn, the brash welled up in my mouth and then I just new I was going to vomit, no matter how I tried to control it, I heaved into the receptacle held by the nurse, tears now rolling down my cheeks, not just due to embarrassment, but also shear fear and concern, if they couldn't get the drugs into me how was I ever going to get better? The Consultant had no option but to abandon the remaining treatment and I was admitted to the day ward awaiting a bed on one of the wards.

Lying alone on the bed, I was consciously aware of the footsteps walking around outside, the occasional laughter of the nurse's discussing their recent escapades and yet although they were only a few feet away, I felt as if I was a million miles away from everyone, unwanted and unpleasant thoughts wandering through my mind.

I was subsequently transferred to Newcastle General Hospital where I would be kept in until my treatment was completed and the anti-sickness medication could be reviewed. The reason for this transfer was the fact that at South Tyneside, there were no oncology beds (beds specifically for cancer patient's) nor oncology trained nurses. When I arrived on ward 38 at Newcastle, I was greeted by a member of the nursing staff and shown around the ward and then to what would be my bed. Later a young doctor came along to prod and poke around and ask the requisite questions that had already been asked numerous times previously, such is life! Unable to do anything about it, this repetitive questioning frustrated me although I could not be bothered to argue. Before I started that obscene treatment again I was commenced on a drip that had the highest dose of Metoclopramide that could be given. The idea was to control the sickness before it started, well; it was some thought if it worked and forgive me for being pessimistic however, was this likely? The Mustine was the most emetogenic (ability to cause vomiting) drug known to medicine for the treatment of malignancy at that time. Therefore, it was decided that my regimen would be changed. The Mustine would be substituted for Cyclophosphamide.

I managed to sleep for the duration of this magic drip and awoke to find a nurse and doctor standing at the bottom of my bed, waiting to administer the toxic chemotherapy. In honesty, with the exception of a few butterflies in the stomach, I did feel relatively relaxed, perhaps because I had only just awoken and didn't have much time to think about the impending treatment. I asked for the orange drink before they started and they looked at me with bewilderment, I'm sure they thought I was crazy. However, there was no way they were starting that treatment without that orange, of that I was certain and more importantly, it was neither of those two who had to endure the bizarre and filthy taste of the drug.

After the treatment I tried sleeping but to no avail and decided to walk along to the day room with my drip (salty water to ensure that I didn't become dehydrated). In the day room the television was on with cricket as the entertainment, some entertainment I don't think. One of the guys,

Tom, greeted me and asked what I was having, *"I think it's called COPP"* I replied, similar to me he retorted and we immediately began to compare notes and it turned out that he also had Hodgkin's disease. He was in his early thirties and was a policeman in Cumbria. He told me that his wife had left him as she couldn't cope with his cancer diagnosis, and I thought that I had problems. Tom and I struck up a good friendship over the coming months.

I clearly remember his optimism at the treatment he was receiving and recall being rather envious of his eternal positivism despite experiencing the same side effects as myself. Later in the evening having attempted some food, my stomach began to gurgle, churn and then erupt as its entire contents were deposited into a large vomit bowl. So much for the anti-sickness drip! The plan then was to try a drug called Lorazepam, the mode of action of this drug would not only knock me out, it would also have an amnesic effect.

Now, have you ever tried sleeping in hospital? Now don't get me wrong I'm not being ageist, but some old men can't half snore. As it turned out I shared a bay on the ward with perhaps a couple of guys who could have represented England at the snoring Olympics. At first it was quite funny, but then it became annoying and sadly, not a great deal can be done about that. Of course there were cubicles on the ward but these were reserved for the more poorly patients, especially those who were dying.

That very situation occurred one night on ward 38. The ward was busier than ever before and the nursing staff appeared to be running around without pause and seemed to be spending an awful lot of time around the old man's bed directly opposite to me. The curtains were secretively drawn around his bed with the bed head light on, the remainder of the ward was in relative darkness as doctor followed doctor behind those curtains, when one nurse went behind the curtains she was soon followed by another. Then, that bed head light was switched off and the doctors and nurses made their way from the curtains but significantly, left the curtains closed. Some while later I was awoken by one of the nurse's closing my curtains, having just closed those adjacent to me. Five minutes afterwards and our curtains were drawn back and there before me was an empty bed, freshly made linen neatly folded and no sign of the little old man who had been the scene of such activity only an hour earlier. Sadly, he had passed away, yet another victim of the friendless cancer. My eyes filled with tears when I realised what had happened and a silent acknowledgement that this cancer was quite capable of claiming me.

Many a night in hospital would be spent in the dayroom, often with the night staff and I do believe it is important to highlight that I had nothing but admiration and praise for these nurses. Seeing what they had to cope with was not the most pleasant job in the world but still, their dedication and uncomplaining approach impressed me immensely.

Interestingly, I had noticed that a number of patients on the ward were not having chemotherapy, they were having a different treatment for their cancer and it was called radiotherapy. It seemed to my inexperienced eye that this was a far easier treatment option than the bloody chemotherapy. Why was that not given to me? I'll make the appropriate investigations on this one and perhaps get the treatment changed, that'll be so much easier and perhaps I can get back to work and also the forthcoming Hawkwind tour. My mind was made up, I want radiotherapy. But how wrong could I be?

Another fellow patient was Steve. Steve had a different type of lymphoma to me, but he was still going through the dreaded chemotherapy and that made us kindred spirits. In addition, he was about my age and therefore we had much in common. Steve was about to finish his chemotherapy and start radiotherapy. Unknown to me at the time, Steve had an aggressive advancing disease that required radiotherapy in addition to chemotherapy. This demonstrated that these lymphomas were not only unpredictable but also indiscriminate.

The Consultant came around later that Friday morning and decided that he wanted to keep me in for observation and monitoring until Monday. However, he didn't mention my request for radiotherapy that I had earlier submitted via the nursing staff and as he left, I felt betrayed. The nurse in question told me that she had mentioned my request to Dr. Sheppard but he dismissed it out of hand as a viable option. Surely an explanation of his rationale might have been in the spirit of good communication.

I suppose if I have one criticism of the medical and nursing fraternity back then was the poor communications. As patients, we were aware that the majority of doctors and nurses were not prepared to confront or even discuss the patient's questions and fears regarding cancer. Peer support at that time was invaluable and I believe it is equally important today as it was then.

Patients essentially need each other as support. Yes, of course we couldn't do without the medical and nursing fraternity. However, Doctors and nurses go off shift and can then forget about work until they are next on duty. The cancer patient simply cannot do that, seven days a week, twenty-four hours of every day, as a patient, you are on duty permanently, with cancer as your main companion. Often I and others would be up most of our nights in hospital, concerned at the uncertainty of the future, comparing notes regarding different experiences and that support was and remains invaluable. What about when you are discharged, out of hospital and back at home, there is also a sense of isolation, that mutual peer support is lost until your next admission. Needless to say, family members are essential, they do everything they can and most often a whole lot more. However, they quite simply are not in the same situation as you and therefore, the mutual support patients give to each other is priceless.

By Saturday morning I was feeling much better, something was obviously having the desired effect. Tom had suggested that we took a walk outside to get the morning paper from a corner shop rather than wait for them appearing on the ward. This we did and as we headed back to the hospital, Tom suggested that we stop and have a pint. This seemed like a reasonable idea to me and so we did. The pub was empty and we sat with a pint of beer passing polite conversation, but as our glasses emptied it seemed that both at the same time we turned and faced each other, our faces becoming ever more flushed with redness and we just knew something strange was happening. Therefore, we returned at haste back to the hospital and onto the ward only to be greeted by the Sister who took one look at us and smirked. *"I know where you two have been"* she exclaimed! We felt like a couple of young schoolchildren having been scolded. The drug Procarbazine is an oral capsule and forms a significant part of our treatment as it is taken for seven days. However, unknown to Tom and me, it interacts with a number of products, including alcohol and causes this facial flushing that we now experienced and although there was no major problem other than this and the fact that alcohol will have a greater effect we did feel like a pair of idiots.

This, the third cycle of treatment was certainly not as bad as the first two. Was this because I was kept in hospital, there'd been a change to the anti-sickness medication or the fact that I was having treatment at the same times as others and had some serious peer support? On Monday, I headed back home feeling much more positive than ever before. When I got home, mam was in the kitchen and when I wandered in there she just smiled at me and looked down at the floor and there in front of me was a delightful little puppy, a cross Labrador/German Sheppard and she was a real beauty. Sheba, as she would be named would be my new companion, a distraction from the thought and worry of cancer and its impending treatment. Unknown to me, mam had made the long travel of approximately fifty miles by public transport, just to buy this puppy for me, while I made my journey home from hospital and as a surprise for my return.

The background nausea was still present and this would remain with me for days to follow but Sheba was good company and a great distraction, in fact Sheba would be a great companion for many years. The future treatments had been planned as an inpatient at Newcastle, and this pleased me greatly as it allowed contact with Tom and the other patients in the same position as me, the mutual support that went hand in hand with that contact was essential, support that only another cancer patient could provide.

Chapter Five

I retired early to bed that night in September and felt at perhaps my lowest ebb since discovering my diagnosis, upset that the doctor had been so brutally explicit regarding my future and bewildered as to what course of action I should now take.

Lost Johnny

It is important to explain something about chemotherapy. Chemo-therapy simply means drug therapy or drug treatment, which means that anyone who has taken any kind of drug has had chemotherapy, but commonly people assume that chemotherapy is always cancer treatment, that's a misconception. Actually the correct term for the treatment used to attack cancer is cytotoxic chemotherapy*; cytotoxic drugs are, in the main the drugs used to treat malignant disease, while cytotoxic simply means poisonous to cells and subsequently the aim of treatment is to destroy cells. However, modern day cytotoxic chemotherapy is a crude form of treatment because, not only does it destroy malignant cells, it also destroys healthy cells too. Therefore, as these healthy cells are affected then there is a point at which the healthy cells drop to a low point just before they begin to recover again, but at that low point, at that moment in time then the chemotherapy patient is more susceptible to infection as the white cells are low, at risk of anaemia as the red cells are low and also susceptible to bleeding and or bruising as the platelet cells are low too.

It was during one of these periods that I picked up an infection and a large boil developed on the left side of my cheek and as my white cell count was low because of the chemotherapy, then the boil was getting bigger and angrier rather than receding and I was started on some antibiotics.

* New drugs, such as hormones and antibodies are increasingly being used.

Additionally, mam was a great believer in the 'good old fashioned' bread poultice and this painful remedy was applied to the side of my cheek and the offending boil but, despite this natural intervention, it made little improvement and on return to hospital, the doctor decided that it needed to be lanced (cut with a surgical blade). This was a painful experience and even today there remains a small scar where the boil was demonstrating just how unforgiving this treatment really was. In addition, and ironically I was desperate to get on with the chemotherapy treatment. Despite the mental anguish and the physical attack on my body, the sooner I could get the treatment behind me the sooner I would be able to move my life forward. Unfortunately, on this occasion and due to this infection I had to wait for the privilege of the next chemical torture. The doctor felt that because of the infection and the low white cell count, then my treatment would be delayed a further week, thus prolonging my personal agony. Living with cancer delivers a number of challenges to the individual on a daily basis and these challenges can often be unexpected, this huge boil on the side of my face was certainly unexpected and it caused me a great deal of distress, both mentally and physically. The simple fact is that you do not earn respect from cancer as a disease; the truth is that it simply fails to respect your individuality. It is a barbaric assault on the human anatomy, physically and mentally.

My mood was once again at particularly low ebb, my thoughts filled with the continued need of more chemotherapy but concerned that I had to wait for it. Soon, I would make a decision, but not necessarily the right one though.

Only days later and my mood changed as I was taken by surprise when I opened the front door to be confronted by the postman. In his hands was a large package addressed to me, Mr John Pattison Junior. I signed for the parcel and rushed inside to find that the package was sent from Aunty Mary and Uncle Jerry in North Carolina, they had sent me some authentic Indian wear, including a couple of head bands, neck beads, books, a waist-coat and a special wallet. On each piece there was a ticket demonstrating that this was hand made by the Cherokee Indians of Ooconaluftee Village in the Great Smokey Mountains of North Carolina in America. Mum had been writing to her sister in America to keep her informed of my condition and treatment, at the same time she had quite innocently mentioned my interest in Native American culture. Aunty Mary is the youngest of my mum's sisters and who had married an American GI after the war and subsequently emigrated to the US. Naturally, I had plenty of time on my hands at present and reading was a good pastime; therefore, I began to browse through the book, 'Bury my heart at Wounded Knee'.

The book was an absolutely fascinating insight into many of the persecutions of the Native American Indians and once started, I found it difficult to put it down. I'd only read a couple of chapters and I felt that one day, I must visit these proud yet, undermined people. Remember, this was way back in 1975, long before people started to collect Indian memorabilia as they do today. More importantly, what had been sent across the Atlantic for me was truly authentic. Many, letters would go back and forward between Aunty Mary and I and many of these would include talk of my desire to visit the Indians. Perhaps one day?

Towards the end of July and just before the chemotherapy was due again, Hawkwind appeared at the Mayfair in Newcastle and I new that I had to be there and indeed I managed to drag myself to the show despite feeling completely washed out and drained of enthusiasm and I had hoped the very presence of the band would rekindle my motivation. Unfortunately, I did not feel terribly well and although the sound was great it proved a very long night such was my ever-present companions, fatigue and the constant feeling of nausea. My resentment of this disease was growing stronger and stronger as it was now interfering with my enjoyment of the mighty Hawkwind and that was unacceptable. Worse was to follow, as much to my disgust a chest infection followed close on the heels of the boil that had scarred my face and which had been surgically opened. This infection forced me into hospital during August, which meant that I had to abandon my plans to travel to Reading to attend the rock festival, which would be headlined by Hawkwind. My lonely persecution was intolerable, isolated by a hidden disease and attacked by its very consequences, deprived of my true joy and passion, Hawkwind.

Frustratingly, having missed the Reading Rock Festival I was further saddened and frustrated to hear the news that apparently there had been some disagreement within the group which had led to a momentary disbandment and therefore, my major concern was that the band would cease to function. In essence, stop providing my direction and motivation. Surely this wouldn't happen, I could only hope. They were, after all my driving force, my inspiration to cope with an infernal situation I had little control over.

To compound my concern about the future and of the worries about Hawkwind splitting, I was still bemused by the fact that some of these guys at Newcastle were having this radiotherapy treatment and I was confused as to why it had not been offered to me. No one had taken the time to explain why I had not been considered for this treatment modality. Of course, there was a perfectly logical explanation that I would learn later.

A few days after my discharge from South Shields hospital, chest infection now behind me, I made my way up to Newcastle for the fourth cycle of delayed chemotherapy; fingers crossed that some of the guys that I'd met on my last admission would also be there. Indeed they were and Tom and I met in the day room.

With me on this admission was Hawkwind, they had recently brought out a new album called 'Warrior on the Edge of Time', truly one of their great works and I had taped it from vinyl onto audiocassette so that I could play it on the portable cassette player I had with me. The first track, Assault and Battery, one of the many all time favourites of mine still to this day and, still played by the band today, had, I thought, a most appropriate first verse. *'Lives of great men all remind us, we may make our lives sublime, and departing leave behind us, footprints in the sands of time'.* Being in the situation I was, facing an uncertain future, so many variables racing through my mind, then this could have been written for me. Now, don't get me wrong I am not for one second, saying that I'm a great man, far from it, more a fact that I was leaving my footprints and nothing else in the sands of time, nothing else to show for my short time on earth. Still, once this fourth cycle of chemotherapy was complete, I headed back to

South Shields to await the arrival of my newfound companions, sickness, lethargy, anorexia and isolation.

In September 1975 I made perhaps one of the most foolish decisions of my young life to that date. Stupidly I decided that four lots of chemotherapy was sufficient for me as I was starting to feel quite well, and therefore in my opinion, there was no need to continue with this chemotherapy which was interfering with my life so drastically, enough was enough. I decided, despite the medical staff calculating that I should have a total of six treatments that four was adequate and I took the decision to stop treatment without consulting them. So, having examined myself and found no lumps, I subsequently gave myself a clean bill of health and therefore, to my silly mind, I had now finished the chemotherapy treatment that had caused so much heartache and agonising side effects. It had altered my perceptions, it had made me bitter and it had prevented me from getting out and about and seeing Hawkwind, so many missed opportunities, so many missed gigs. As the disease had controlled me for so long, it was about time I took some control back and foolishly I failed to attend my next hospital appointment and even when a reminder came through the post a few days later, I ignored it as I felt that I had been living my life around the cancer, that, in my view, was not right and in ignorance I thought I would put the cancer experience right behind me! It was as easy as that, or was it?

The medical staff at hospital were obviously concerned that I had foolishly failed to attend for my scheduled appointment and the penultimate chemotherapy that would have been due at that time. It was less than six weeks from completing my chemotherapy (or so I thought), when one evening after tea, I was sitting at home with my family, still trying to get my head around the notion that I had cancer and trying to be optimistic that it would not return, when there was a loud knock on the door.

Imagine my amazement to open the door and find my family doctor standing there larger than life, and he was a larger than life individual, he must have weighed at least 25 stone and he immediately went into a rambling narration regarding the importance of starting the treatment again, because if I didn't, I would be organising my own funeral. Not only was he, in my opinion, an incompetent doctor, he was also inept at communication skills. What a bloody cheek coming to my front door and talking to me about funerals, but not just any funeral, my funeral. In hindsight of course, he did have my best intention at heart I suppose, although I didn't see it at the time and I may have been blinkered by his previous ineptitude, treating me for depression.

I retired early to bed that night in September and felt at perhaps my lowest ebb since discovering my diagnosis, upset that the doctor had been so brutally explicit regarding my future and bewildered as to what course of action I should now take. What should I do? During that endless night, I felt dismally lonely and confused, but also very tearful and without a friend in the world who could advise me of the correct course of action, I was annoyed by the attempts to stifle my exposure to the truth and wanted control of my destiny or at least some say in it. Now that I had control, it was not very easy or pleasant. Equally, this was a no win situation, I consciously did not discuss these, my most deep and sincere emotions with my parents simply because I knew the hurt they too would share at my anguish. I was not convinced that I could honestly tolerate the onslaught of those drugs again and the inevitable consequences they brought with them and if I explained this to my parents they would be destroyed. However, with little sleep that night I think that I probably matured overnight and hesitantly decided the following morning that my future could only be guaranteed if I completed that despicable chemotherapy. Surely, if the experts were recommending this barbaric treatment then it must be necessary, they wouldn't put anyone through that just for the sake of it.

I returned, reluctantly to the Hospital on Thursday for my fifth course of those destructive drugs acknowledging that once again, I would be living my life around that cancer and no longer in control. I wasn't sure if the medical staff were now making an example of me because I had foolishly decided that four treatments were sufficient and they insisted that I have my scheduled treatment at the Diagnostic Centre at South Tyneside as an outpatient, rather than as an inpatient at Newcastle. Then again, perhaps I was being somewhat paranoid. At times it felt as if everything was conspiring against me and nothing appeared to go the way the medical fraternity had expected, or was this just my interpretation? How could you receive a treatment aimed at ridding your very body of a cancer invasion and yet, that chemical poison damaged all in its path, my mind included!

Sadly, the fear and anxiety led me to feel nauseated even before I entered the premises, a feeling I knew all too well. Clearly in my mind, I remember feeling the sharp prick of the needle breach my skin and almost immediately, the cold toxic substance being pushed along the syringe and into my fragile veins. Emotionally, I could not face anymore of this, my mind was just buzzing with the fear and knowledge of what the consequence of this chemotherapy would be. Once again, as had happened some months earlier the Consultant stopped the treatment with little of the intended drugs delivered. It was not just his compassion and sincerity, it was also the empathy of the nursing sister that made me feel even more upset and tearful. My body trembled, my head was spinning and I wept uncontrollably.

Once again, I was transferred to Newcastle General Hospital and to the welcome embrace of ward 38 where a regimen of intravenous fluids and a similar cocktail of drugs that had worked quite well on my first admission were being prepared. The chemotherapy treatment would not be given until the following day as it was now early evening. I was kept in hospital for a couple of days following the chemotherapy and deliberately did not come out of the cubicle for fear of meeting anyone I had previously hoped I would see again. Such was my mental state that I was not ready for peer support and their genuine empathy. Dr. Sheppard came in to see me on the Monday morning and told me I'd be going home and that in view of my inability to tolerate the cytotoxic chemotherapy, this fifth course would be my last.

However, sitting on the side of my bed Dr. Sheppard told me that it was highly unlikely that the amount of treatment that I had already received would be sufficient to control this highly aggressive lymphoma. He looked straight into my eyes and said with conviction, *"there is less chance of getting rid of the illness than previously thought, but we must try"*. Therefore, he had decided on an alternative treatment, one that was gentler but would complement what had already been given. I admired his honesty and asked for some clarification on what this alternative was.

The new regimen would include some oral chemotherapy tablets called Cyclophosphamide taken for 14 days (previously given as an intravenous agent). In addition, I would be required to take more steroids. But most importantly, another component would be a drug called Bleomycin and which was administered as an injection into the muscle. The plan was to have the injections twice each week for two weeks.

What did I have to lose, it didn't sound too harsh and what's more the Consultant had said that if I felt up to it, then I could return to work and have the on-site doctor administer the injections. To my frustration and consternation, the doctor at Readheads Shipyard decided he wanted nothing to do with this chemotherapy and it was left to my family doctor to give. The treatment wasn't too bad in comparison to what I had previously been given and it did allow me to get back to work, which was important to me. That said, such was my desire to get back to work that once home at the end of the working day, I simply had no energy for anything else and my social life was none existent. The intramuscular injections where bloody painful and meant you couldn't sit for about an hour afterwards, but this treatment only lasted for two weeks after which I would then have a four week break before commencing the next course.

Thankfully, after two months of this most unusual of treatments and after a physical examination, no lymph nodes could be detected and my bloods were normal, Dr. Sheppard felt that that should be enough. Therefore, I'm told go and enjoy what it is that I wanted to enjoy, no questions about that one was there, Hawkwind. So, from diagnosis in the May, the barbarism of those investigations, the persecution of Minnie Rippiton and the psychological devastation of the unknown, the betrayal of being undermined in respect to the attempts to keep my diagnosis secret, the trials and tribulations of dealing with chemotherapy, the euphoria and then the depressive decline of accepting the knowledge that your very existence was always under threat, to what I foolishly intended to be the end of treatment in September and at last, now the treatment is finished; perhaps I can now put this whole chapter of my life behind me. What a relief and yet I felt somewhat isolated, gone was the safety net of the hospital, yes, I'd be back and forward for check ups but not the intensive contact I'd been used too.

The good thing was that Hawkwind were planning yet another tour and guess who would be there? You'd better believe it, even though it would mean another trip to London as Newcastle was not on the itinerary.

I felt that it was most important to get back to work, purely and simply to normalise my life, but to prove that the cancer was not going to dictate what I could and could not do in my life. On my return to Readheads ship-yard I was asked to make an appointment with one of the training officers. In his office I'm told that the management had decided that because of my serious condition (the posh term for cancer, or the fear of adults to call it cancer) then it wasn't practical for me to return to welding and therefore I was allocated to the plating shed. This job was cleaner and also presented less toxic fumes.

My time in the shipyards was a pleasant one; the industry was full of some weird and wonderful characters. People such as Mickey F****** Broon so named because that between every other word he used was the 'F' word. He called me F****** shite hawk, his reason? He likes the hawks and he's full of F****** shite. I really have no idea were he got his rationale from but he was a harmless guy. Jimmy the carthorse, my previous fore-man (the one who caught me asleep in the cofferdams) came up to me to ask how I was. I think he felt bad about the verbal rollicking he'd given me that day and said, "*you should have said you were poorly*". Actually I felt quite sorry for Jimmy that day. Word had quickly spread throughout this small shipyard of my diagnosis and many of the older guys in the shipyards made an effort to come and speak with me that afternoon and that was important, even those guys who hardly new me. In such a small shipyard there was a great sense of camaraderie.

The management at Readheads shipyard were very supportive. If I wanted or needed time off work, then I only had to say the word. It was a good time, a time when life appeared to be getting back to normal, or so I thought and always in the back of my mind was the inevitable fear of cancer, how long would I be well? Soon, very soon, I would have that answer.

In the interim, I had to put those dreaded thoughts to the back of my mind and get on with life. Fishing would also prove to be an escape mechanism, Neil, also from the yards was a good friend and we'd spend many a night sitting on the end of the rocks at Marsden fishing. More importantly, when I'd go to his house, his wife, Jean would be there. Now Jean was a nurse and I had developed a huge admiration for the work that they did and I felt this was something I would like do. Of course, at that time I had no qualifications, nor was I going to leave a relatively well-paid job in the shipyard for a career in nursing, but talk of nursing excited and interested me, oh what it would be to have a fulfilling and satisfying career.

Our fishing expeditions would become regular occurrences; I think it's referred to as escapism. I vividly remember one night sitting on the rock edges peering out into the black wilderness way out to sea and seeing a shooting star diving toward the earth. No need to explain here what I wished for that night, was this an omen?

Between treatments, Robbo and I would spend many nights at the City Hall in Newcastle seeing a whole host of different bands; it helped marginalize the deviation from normality and gave me a sense of acceptance, doing the things that normal teenagers do. This behaviour would continue even after treatment too and I was delighted that I could resume this way of life.

Christmas 1975 and I felt better than I had for sometime and at least I was getting out and about with some of the lads. I knew that there eagle eyes were constantly focussed on me and ready to protect me should the need arise, although importantly, it never ever was necessary. More and more people would come up to me and ask how I was, even those that I didn't know too well and I appreciated this, a recognition on my behalf that people were indeed, well intentioned and that the world wasn't such a bad place after all. It was around this juncture in time that I realised what I'd missed over the past couple of years and now enjoyed the social scene and felt quite optimistic.

Unfortunately, my optimism was short lived and, mid way through April 1976 and I began to feel unwell, only a few months after finishing treatment the tell tale signs began to appear. Lumps in the axilla (armpit) could indicate only one thing, its back! I had no other option but to get in touch with the hospital and bring forward my appointment. The night sweats had once again started and I had specific chest pains. The Bleomy-cin and Cyclophosphamide had failed to halt the determined advancement of this obstinate cancer. What would there approach be now? Would they have another approach? Perhaps as a believer in fate, then I had to accept that my existence was not intended to be a long one and that eventually this cancer would ultimately claim my life.

At hospital, the obligatory blood test and physical examination confirmed that the cancer was again becoming active and that further treatment would be required. At least, I thought to myself, they were not giving up, even though I had an inherent fear of the treatment they proposed.

I am told that there is a swollen gland in the left axilla and at least a couple in the groin. This represented a second relapse in the face of active treatment and as if they hadn't learned anything about communication, my mam and dad are taken to one side and told that it will now prove more difficult to control what is obviously an aggressive lymphoma, it also means that the original chances of a 50% survival rate can be reduced even further, although no specific figure was offered. Foolishly, I had taken the decision to get a second tattoo and it was soon afterwards that I had relapsed. Therefore, mam had no hesitation in blaming the tattoo for the recurrence of the cancer, although there was no evidence to support this. During our discussions many years later mam told me that it would not be uncommon for her to cry uncontrollably and without warning such was her and my father's consternation and worry at the future and the fear of losing their son.

The evidence in relation to the different drugs available to the Consultant means that the first drugs chosen to treat the cancer obviously have the best chance of getting rid of the disease once and for all even though initially, my parents where told that my chances of survival were approximately fifty fifty. This was a guarded statement as I had such extensive disease and back in the early 70's, Hodgkin's disease remained a killer. Mam and dad were also told that this percentage would naturally diminish if I did not respond to the selected drug cocktail; this is called a relapse or disease progression and I now faced another relapse. Subsequent drugs chosen after the first selection have less chance of destroying the malignant cells.

It was now that I expressed abhorrence at being confronted by more chemotherapy and really did not want this. To this end, I informed the registrar who had informed me that the disease was once again active that I could not guarantee that I would complete the planned treatment, but when the registrar who saw me said I'd be going to Newcastle for treatment, that meant only one thing to me, I was going to get radiotherapy even though he never actually came out and said that. Well, I'd seen the others tolerate this treatment when I was at Newcastle and it appeared to be absent of side effects, so I agreed to attend ward 38 again the following day. It really is amazing that at times we hear what it is that we want to hear and to the exclusion of everything else. What's more surprising is the fact that we actually believe it too. This was one of those very examples.

On the ward and things where really no different than six month earlier. The same nursing staff but no familiar faces from a patient's perspective. My bed was at the top end of the ward next to an old guy sleeping in his bed and who didn't look terribly well. Along came the junior doctor to ask the now familiar questions and then proceeded to tell me that the chemotherapy would start later in the afternoon. *"Hang on there"*, I said, *"I'm not here for chemotherapy, I'm having radiotherapy"*. The doctor looked bewildered, checked the medical notes, was somewhat confused and trotted off to the office.

Almost immediately along came Sid, one of the staff nurses that by now, I knew very well. Sid tried to explain that chemotherapy had been planned for me and that because of the fact that my cancer was quite wide spread throughout the body, then radiotherapy really wasn't an option. Now I was upset, I felt betrayed and let down, if that's all that's on offer then thanks but no thanks, I am not having more chemotherapy to go through all that that brings with it. I can recall quite clearly that Sid was taken aback, but he then carried on telling me that this was my only option. But my mind was made up; I would accept no more of this shit (the treatment that is)!

Sid sat on the bedside and spoke slowly and concisely, thinking of his next sentence, "*if you don't have treatment you may not survive this cancer*", and his blunt but honest words echoed around my head. In the first instance I felt angry, easy for him to sit there and say that, its not him stuck with this bloody cancer inside. However, very quickly I felt guilty at having those thoughts, he was only trying to help and it certainly could not have been easy to sit there beside me, not knowing how I would respond. At this point, I made perhaps the most important decision of my life. "*I am not having chemotherapy and, if I have to die, then that's it*". My decision was final! And yet strangely, I did not find this decision a difficult one to make; on the contrary, I felt a huge burden lift from my shoulders. Surprisingly, even to me, I remained very calm but I do remember feeling sad for my family, not myself.

It's difficult trying to convey this concept to anyone because people may say, you'd cling to every opportunity, grasp any chance you have, and yes of course some people would. However, the emotional turmoil, the debilitating nausea, the gut wrenching vomiting and the psychological confusion is beyond comprehension, the depressive isolation intolerable. Anticipating how you're going to feel before it's even started was something I felt was not an option I was prepared to accept.

Sid however, not to be beaten, asked if we could discuss things in a more private setting and although I was adamant that I was not having chemotherapy I agreed to his request. Sid did not try and directly persuade me to have more chemotherapy, instead he spoke of how he himself could not even begin to imagine what the treatment was like and I respected his honesty and approach. He also spoke of my family and the affect my decision would have on them. Ultimately, Sid in some psychological process convinced me that chemotherapy was the route to take and so I very reluctantly agreed to further treatment. I'm unsure if Sid realised exactly the monumental change of heart he had instigated that day, but one thing is for certain, he inspired me to continue and I do not believe many others could have done that. Sadly, many years later Sid would leave nursing and take up social work and I'd never see him again. Nursing's loss was certainly social works gain. I often wonder what might have been if Sid had not been on duty that day, I do not believe that many other nurses back in 1976 would have talked so openly and honestly about death as Sid did with me. If you happen to read this Sid, I owe you big time and thanks.

I believe that in many regards, some nurses and indeed, some doctors working in the demanding field of cancer care become therapeutic friends to patients, but it's difficult to see sometimes where this relationship starts, where does it end or, does it ever end? What is certain is the fact that without these therapeutic friends, cancer patients would be lost.

Subsequently for me, it was chemotherapy time again. The dosages where changed from what had previously been given due to my inability to both physically and mentally cope with the wrath of chemotherapy. Some of the specific drugs used now would be changed from what I'd previously been given as it was pointless giving the same drugs again when the disease had become so active so very quickly.

The junior doctor tells me that before more treatment is given I require a blood transfusion. As a consequence of all the treatment and all of the subsequent needles, it was becoming increasingly more difficult to locate good veins. Therefore, the needle was sited in my foot as the veins in my upper limbs were proving somewhat unresponsive so after a third attempt, the feet were thought to be a better option. This of course, restricted my mobility and I was left stuck lying on top of the bed.

Unfortunately for me despite a different cocktail of drugs, the treatment was pretty similar to what I had received earlier in the year and the side effects were just as I'd remember them, inexplicable! Time seemed to go nowhere; in fact it almost lasted forever. One day simply merged into the next with little respite from the nausea and general lethargy.

Chemotherapy had started again on 28th May 1976 almost one year exactly since diagnosis, and treatment was planned as regular as possible depending upon the recovery of my healthy cells. The expectation was that the chosen chemotherapy treatment on this occasion would be administered at ten day intervals, although from time to time, ten days was simply not enough time for my healthy cells to recover and I would be delayed a further week, this of course was depressing as it meant I could see little end to my unwanted nightmare. These deferrals were essential otherwise the chemotherapy could have quite easily taken my life from me as with a reduced white cell count my immune system could not and would not function adequately if faced with any opportunistic infection. Of course I had some difficulty understanding this concept and I was very frustrated as these delays simply prolonged my agony, while all I wanted to do was get on with it so that hopefully I could put whatever treatment was planned behind me.

That troublesome mental anxiety would be compounded by the development of shingles between treatments. I awoke one morning to discover this weird rash covering the left side of my torso and boy, was it painful. Mam insisted that this was a matter for the hospital as I'd had a previous drug reaction and therefore, off I trot to the Diagnostic Centre at South Shields. It would also cause a temporary halt to the chemotherapy, not to mention the significant sharp stinging pain all down my left side, which seemed unresponsive to simple painkillers. My sleep pattern was not the best at the majority of times, but this shingles infection (viral infection similar to chicken pox and which invades nerve endings) was causing additional problems, my mind was now in overdrive thinking that this nightmare was never going to end. What the hell was happening to my body? and when, if ever, would I regain control? Patients receiving chemotherapy naturally become immunocompromised (reduced ability to fight infection) and any opportunistic infection has the potential to capitalise on a weak and vulnerable immune system and invade. I was given some medication and told to restrict myself to the house, some quality of life that was. In many respects and in hindsight, I probably got off quite lightly with the shingles; some patients are far more debilitated than I ever was. To me, the biggest problem was the suppression of your normal thoughts, the inactivity of rationalisation.

The weeks came and went, each day merged into the next and time was of little relevance any longer; the hospital setting became my second home and the staff part of my extended family. Despite that supportive network, and of course, not forgetting my family, chemotherapy treatment was no easier to accept or receive. An uneasy anxiety, a predictable fear leading up to each and every treatment, knowing fine well that following on from the chemotherapy my body no longer had any respect for what it was I wanted it to do, it had a mind all of its own, controlled of course by those life saving drugs. It was if your body was bereft of vitality, the vigour drained from within by an unrelenting attack. The known consequences made it far less easy to accept, the waiting and anticipation of the side effects made life intolerable for a teenager in the 70's, I was no longer 'normal'. I felt as though I was becoming a submissive entity with nothing more than a silent voice. My views, feelings or wishes were never considered and although my best interest was always at the forefront, what about my concerns, my needs, what about my identity? Eventually, some five months down the line and the infernal cocktail of treatment was thankfully complete.

However, now that the treatment was once again terminated, I'm planning my return to full time employment and more importantly, the next Hawkwind concert. Indeed, September 1976 at Newcastle City Hall would prove a spectacular event with an equally amazing light show to match the fantastic space rock that only Hawkwind could provide. Additionally, and as the band's tour was still in full swing around the country, then after this show I was determined to ensure I saw them again. Therefore, once again I arranged the necessary payment for the scheduled performance of Hawkwind at the famous Hammersmith Odeon the following month. My plan was to make my way to the big city and demonstrate my support for the band. Subsequently, less than a week later that all-important ticket arrived making me wonder, was life finally returning to normal? It wouldn't be too long before I got the answer, and not the answer I expected.

Back at work and Readheads shipyard in South Shields was now preparing to close down and transfer its workforce to other yards along the River Tyne and I was no exception. I was allocated a place at Swan Hunters at Wallsend and the day I walked into the new department, my hair was still absent, although it was slowly starting to come back in. One guys comment to another colleague was just a little too loud and I overheard his sarcastic criticism of my strange hairstyle. I was hurt and offended by this and felt that this was not the kind of area I wished to work in, although sadly, I had no option. In addition, and more despairingly I had already decided a few days earlier to cancel my planned trip to London as I was now beginning to recognise those tell tale signs of recurrence and the associated feelings that went hand in hand with them. I knew that it would be impossible to make the long journey to London feeling the way I did, tired and emotionally on the edge, those drenching night sweats informing me that my unwanted accomplice was yet again returning. Sitting in my bedroom, staring at my unused ticket for the Hammersmith Odeon left me tearful and frustrated, and once again wondering what the immediate future had in store for me.

My next appointment was a few weeks away and in all honesty I should have contacted the hospital to bring it forward as I knew exactly what was occurring deep within my body. Feeling depressed and isolated I trudged along to my scheduled appointment early in November 1976 terrified like never before as to what management strategy might be initiated. Frustratingly, it is my first clinic appointment since completing the last lot of chemotherapy and although deep down I knew what was happening, I paradoxically prayed that I would get a clean bill of health. It's crazy how as individuals we try to convince ourselves that things are going well and I desperately wanted to be well, sadly and as expected my worst fears were realised, a third relapse and which came as no surprise at all. It is the worst news I could wish to hear and I'm told that the chemotherapy has only had a partial response, a large lymph node quite evident in my right axilla and that more treatment would be required. I was, perhaps for the first time in my life, speechless, gutted, bewildered and confused as to where we go from here as I had pinned so much hope on the last chemotherapy that I had reluctantly accepted and my immediate response was one of anger.

I now felt more vulnerable than ever before, I also felt that perhaps, as a believer in destiny that my end was in sight. Perhaps my biggest problem was the fact that as a young man I had always chosen not to discuss much of my illness or even its savage side effects with anyone. Was this though an unconscious decision by me knowing how difficult my family had found the diagnosis and the uncertain future it bestowed upon me? But then, was it a paradox that when my parents agreed with the Consultant at diagnosis, not to inform me of that disease, it was partly their own inability to accept the cancer diagnosis and how they could address my questions should I ask the inevitable, that being, my own mortality. I'd always chosen to go to hospital on my own, now I desperately needed someone, no one was there and I wandered off home in a stupefied demeanour. This was a third relapse and had dire consequences.

Once again, I began to acknowledge and yet at the same time, question my own mortality, would I ever be in a position to see my own children grow up, would I be able to see Sheba develop? The concerns as to whether life would end soon, the never-ending worry as to exactly what fate had in store for me as an individual! Questions and concerns that rolled around my mind almost constantly, and yet, no other person could offer any answers. Simply, this was part of life's wonderful tapestry and my fate was woven into it.

Compounding the predicament was the fact that I kept my fears and concerns to myself. My fragile emotions and worries would belong to me and me alone as I felt that my parents and sister did not deserve to have to share this burden. I knew how difficult my family were finding the whole ordeal and subsequently I kept this personal turmoil inside as a protective factor in favour of my family. Of course, in hindsight that was not the thing to do as I struggled constantly to deal with the fears and strange dilemmas that would invade my mind on a daily basis, questions my sub-conscious would ask of me, questions I would refuse to answer. I had no answers to the myriad of self posed questions my mind asked of me and in reality it would have helped if I'd shared some of that responsibility, after all, this wasn't just my cancer, it was affecting the entire family and they deserved the opportunity to help me, yet in absolute naivety, I denied them that chance and also myself the support that it would have brought with it. I suppose in essence, the fact remains that there is no preparation for the fight against cancer, whether it is you the individual or a member of your family. No one person can say this is what you should do; it remains the ultimate discovery of your inner self. A discovery that is made as you travel the lonely and unpredictable road of the cancer journey and I was no exception.

Chapter Six

Christmas 1976 was without doubt, the worst Christmas of my entire life. My get up and go, got up of its own volition and went, leaving me bereft of vigour, drained of enthusiasm, in the depths of despair and persecuted by an illness I could not see and more importantly, had no control over, that said, I now had respect for this potential killer disease that was proving rather difficult to eliminate.

Brainbox Pollution

It was around this time that I met Dr. Bozzino, a Consultant Oncologist and Dr. Atkinson, a specialist registrar, both of whom would prove very important factors in my life as between them, they took over my care and management. The reason for this was that Dr. Sheppard had accepted a new Consultant post down under in Australia, although until his departure, I would still see him from time to time, as would my parents!

It was now that the medical fraternity proposed that radiotherapy should be utilised as my treatment, but my understanding of the situation was that in an ideal world radiotherapy would not be the most suitable treatment for me. Yes, I had bulky disease in the mediastinum (chest) but also some disseminated disease elsewhere and therefore; systemic treatment in the form of chemotherapy would be required. Significantly, I had already made up my mind and the medical team new fine well what my response to a different kind of chemotherapy would be. There is only so much one man can take, and although many may see it as my weakness, I'm afraid I simply could not have taken anymore of the infernal solution, I could not contemplate more chemotherapy and the debilitating effects it was having on me and taking away almost permanently my individuality, at least that was my perception, these were my inner thoughts.

Therefore, I was asked to make my way once again to Newcastle General Hospital to get prepared for radiotherapy. However, I was also told that this treatment would be delivered as an outpatient and that an ambulance would take me back and forth to Newcastle each day, Monday to Friday for five weeks.

Radiotherapy is a treatment that is given to localised disease, that is to say, it is aimed at getting rid of cancer in one specific area, whereas chemotherapy is a systemic treatment, it would get into every nook and cranny of the human form. That was the main reason why radiotherapy had not been considered for my condition before now; they needed a treatment that would attack the widespread nature of my cancer. But of course at the time, I did not have that information. Why on earth this was never explained to me before, well, that's anyone's guess; it would have made perfect sense and perhaps softened my anger at not being considered for radiotherapy before now. From a cynical viewpoint I wondered if they thought that as a young adolescent I wasn't capable of comprehending this simple explanation?

Radiotherapy is given in a similar fashion to a simple X-Ray; of course there is a much larger dose of radiation used. However, it isn't just a case of aiming a beam of radiation at the desired area; special precautions had to be taken. In the first instance special metal blocks were made in order to protect my lungs as the damaging rays of ionising radiation could cause permanent damage to those organs. This type of radiotherapy was called mantle irradiation and delivered treatment from the mandible down to the diaphragm. The first dose of radiotherapy was an absolute breeze taking literally a few minutes to deliver. I had my skin marked, similar to a Cherokee brave so that the radiographers new where to position me on the couch for subsequent treatments, 23 in total, one treatment each day, Monday to Friday.

Of course like most of the treatments for cancer the side effects were often more potent than the actual disease itself and radiotherapy was no exception, as it would also damage healthy cells as it destroyed malignant cells too. I was having mediastinal radiotherapy; that is to say, most of my chest was in the treatment field. Unknown to me, the treatment, similar to chemotherapy, would have specific side effects which would affect my quality of life and it would prove not to be without side effects as I had wrongly assumed.

It had been me, who had persistently argued and insisted on having radiotherapy having seen all of those other chaps receive that form of treatment at Newcastle. It had seemed free of side effects, but how wrong I would be. The first three weeks of radiotherapy went without any problem, however, like chemotherapy treatment, radiotherapy also affects healthy cells and so the treatment began to take its savage toll on my young body.

At first, these side effects crept up on me very gradually. Firstly, the tiredness left me so fatigued that I would feel the need to sleep for at least a couple of hours on my return from hospital. Secondly, my throat became hoarse and I had difficulty swallowing. Soon afterwards the sickness started and proved just as difficult as the chemotherapy-induced sickness to control.

The plan was for twenty-three treatments consisting of a total of 3436 rads (measure of radiation), to the chest and neck, with a final booster of 500 rads to the right axilla, the area that refused to succumb to the usual powerful constraints of chemotherapy. At Newcastle where the radiotherapy was given the small waiting area was crammed wall to wall with patient's waiting to receive their treatment, a constant production line which is exactly what you do not want when your feeling grotty, tired and just wanting to be anywhere other than hospital. At times I felt trapped, if I died then at least that would be a release, but instead I'm alive and stuck with this burden of cancer.

Christmas 1976 was without doubt, the worst Christmas of my entire life. My get up and go, got up of its own volition and went, leaving me bereft of vigour, drained of enthusiasm, in the depths of despair and persecuted by an illness I could not see and, more importantly, had no control over, But, I now had even more respect for this potential killer disease that was proving rather difficult to eliminate. To make matters worse I found that my appetite was perhaps the worse thing affected, perhaps due to the constant feeling of nausea. Everything I tried to eat tasted like soggy cardboard and my mum was obviously concerned and tried all kinds of tempting dishes with little success. She even went out and bought the build up drink Complan to try and tempt my taste buds. Now correct me if I'm wrong here but, if someone is not eating then the last thing there going to want is some bland, tasteless unappetising drink that was supposed to be delivering the nutritional support I was lacking. Complan was exactly that, bland and tasteless and it was not for me.

To make matters worse, as the radiotherapy exerted its effect on the disease in my chest, the pains I experienced where crippling. They would come on at the most inopportune moment and caused me to freeze with discomfort and fear, fear that this was the progression of cancer. Although I had been prescribed strong painkillers, these had unwanted side effects and caused my head to spin as if I had consumed a bottle of 'Jim Beam' (my favourite tipple). Even the painkillers had bloody side effects. The pain would be worse at night when I was alone, the pain exacerbated by the silence and darkness. I felt lost and persecuted by an uninvited entity inside and which refused to leave me.

Radiotherapy continued through until 28th January 1977 and what was a freezing winter with plenty of snow on the ground. Trying to motivate myself, I remember going for short walks in the snow and I think in all honesty it was at this stage that I felt sorrier for myself than at any other moment in time. I was aware that all of the lads would be out enjoying themselves, and although they regularly called in during the day to see me, night time was a different ball game. As you would expect, I was not eating and I began to lose weight that concerned not only mam and dad, but also the hospital. I believe that there was some consideration of stopping the radiotherapy at this point, but that never happened.

During the radiotherapy treatment you were not allowed to wash the area being treated (irradiated) and subsequently, I developed a large 'tide' mark around the back of my neck. Additionally, I had not had a bath for the entire duration of treatment and my hair had not been washed for the same period of time, instead you were allowed to use talcum powder both on your skin and your hair. Of course, I'm sure you can appreciate that this does not work the same as good old soap and water. I felt filthy and dear knows what I smelled like, although in fairness, no one ever gave me the slightest inclination that there was a problem. It was the time of the good old 'Brut' aftershave adverts on television and Christmas had brought me my fair share of the smelly cologne. Therefore, each and every morning religiously during the radiotherapy days, I would splash it all over as someone once so famously said.

On completion of this particular treatment modality I had to wait a further fourteen days afterwards, as the radiation was still effective on my skin for that duration. Eventually though, that day arrived and my mum had filled the most enticing bath I'd ever wished for, tentatively I climbed in and I lay there till the water became cold. Despite my long and relaxing soak, the tide mark remained for some weeks thereafter and this was the source of much ridicule by my mam and she made it her business to tell everyone about the now famous tide mark around my neck. Despite the seriousness and gravity of the situation it was good to laugh, especially at myself, in fact, it was essential and a good coping mechanism too.

As the weeks progressed I began to get stronger and stronger and began to get the urge to return to work. I also began to dream about visiting America and the Indian reservation at Ooconaluftee village. I had been keeping in regular contact with Aunty Mary and the offer to visit was permanently on the table.

My hospital visits continued at monthly intervals, monitoring my blood counts and not forgetting the physical examination. As the time progressed during these, my formative years, I matured rather quickly and appreciated that life was not only important, but also precious. I soon deduced that for the majority of people they did not respect the sanctity of life. This was my conclusion, seeing individual after individual abuse themselves and, I had no doubt, had illness not intervened, then I too would have been just another who took life for granted. I was slowly but surely earning more and more respect for this cancer, but equally accepting that it was teaching me a very valuable lesson about life. Enjoy it while you can, it won't be there forever, or should I say, we won't be here forever.

Things went ok for some weeks, but soon things took an almost expected downward plunge. March 1977, only five weeks after completion of the radiotherapy I discovered a lump (swollen lymph node) under my left arm and new exactly what this meant, progression of the lymphoma and more treatment. This represented a fourth relapse. Admittedly, I was feeling very low and although at times I visualised that perhaps my life was not destined to be a long one, I did not want to allow the depressive feelings to take over my mind and again my motivation proved to be Hawkwind. Now, I think it is important to highlight that my family were vitally significant in my life. Hawkwind however, allowed me the opportunity for escapism and distraction. Additionally, I loved, and still do their music, there was and is no equal to Hawkwind. Unfortunately, as much as I could have done with seeing Hawkwind at this juncture in my illness they were not around, they were touring Europe and I was definitely unable to access them this time, my thoughts turned to when I would see them again, my thoughts turned to whether I would see the again, my mood following peaks and troughs of uncontrollable dimensions.

Some twelve months earlier, I would have shuddered at the thought of more chemotherapy and the potential dangers that it brought with it. But today, I was determined that I had so much to live for. My family were right behind me and supported me to the very best of their ability. They felt my pain and shared my anguish as if it were theirs. I knew I had their undivided support, but equally, I knew that not to accept further treatment would be the ultimate self-destruct that may also destroy them.

Unbeknown to me, my parents were spoken too by Dr. Sheppard and told that control of this aggressive Hodgkin's lymphoma was not likely. From a medical perspective, it was only a matter of time, but I would succumb to this unresponsive cancer. The plan therefore, from this moment in time was palliative chemotherapy (treatment that had little or no side effects, but designed to control symptoms and extend my life, not cure it). The decision had apparently already been made without my consent, nothing new there then! However, here is the ethical dilemma, if I'd been told of the current situation, would I have accepted the offer of further chemotherapy? I suggest not, there is only so much any one individual can take and in my eyes I'd taken it.

One important factor in the history of my illness is the use of complementary therapy. My mum had been reading about this wonder root called Ginseng and the significant improvement it could make to the human body. The book she had read claimed that the root could improve life and rid the body of many conditions and ailments. It was now that she went out and bought a supply of this herb. Each day I would regimentally take one capsule and even to this day, mum still thinks this herbal root played a significant role in my recovery. Who can argue?

When I returned to work following the radiotherapy I struggled to complete a full five days and at times I completed less than a full week's work. Management were good and on the whole very supportive, their approach was, come in when you can get in. I truly appreciated this and made every endeavour to get into work at every opportunity. My tiredness was marked but my thoughts were now focussed on the next Hawkwind tour, where would that be and would I manage to get there?

At my next clinic appointment, Dr. Bozzino and Dr. Atkinson, both of whom I had become good friends with over the months, saw me. Dr. Bozzino speaks to me directly, as a person, giving me the time to ask specific questions. Now I'm not saying that Dr. Sheppard hadn't spoken to me as a person, he did and he was an excellent doctor. I just felt that he collaborated too much with my parents about my disease and my management. After all, this was my disease and I felt he attempted, although well intentioned, to take it away from me.

Dr. Bozzino was an articulate and pleasant gentleman who made me feel very relaxed. His time was my time and importantly, he made time to ensure that I had asked all the questioned that I needed. His eternal optimism was heart-warming even if he knew something I didn't. Dr. Atkinson would always have a special place in my heart for the reasons you will soon discover. He is a tall Englishman with an excellent disposition, someone who enjoys a good laugh, someone I could relate too, empathetic and professional. I would develop the utmost respect for both men.

At this consult they told me that I'd had a fair response to the radiotherapy, but, there was this persistent node under my arm and some deep para-aortic lymph nodes (deep in the abdomen) which needed to be targeted by some treatment, nodes that had not been treated by the radiotherapy. What they meant was palliative chemotherapy to improve my quality of life, something that Dr. Sheppard had already discussed with my parents. Whether Dr. Bozzino and Dr. Atkinson were aware of that collusion I'm not sure, I prefer to believe that they didn't, but honestly suspect they did.

I'm told that the weekly injections are almost free from side effects. Now that is certainly something that impresses me immediately, was this possible, no side effects? Why did I not get this drug from the offset? The reason, well, of course it's intended to resolve some of my symptoms and push the disease into the background, not to cure it.

At that same appointment, I was asked to go for a coffee until the drug can be manufactured in pharmacy and I'm happy to oblige as I'm getting lots of information from these two chaps and most importantly I'm being involved in the decision making process. Obviously, they hadn't had the drug made on the assumption that I'd accept the treatment, as had previously been the situation. Therefore, around to the WRVS coffee bar and approximately an hour or so later one of nurses comes looking for me to say that Dr. Bozzino is now ready for me. Dr. Atkinson is away off to see another patient and I was subsequently whisked straight back into the consulting room that I now know so very well. Dr. Bozzino has a butterfly needle in the back of my hand before I know it and taped in position. The drug, Vinblastine, is administered in no time at all, the butterfly is removed and I'm on my way home.

Over the next three month I would attend the outpatient department to see either Dr. Atkinson or Dr.Bozzino and to have Vinblastine, 10mg. The dose was dependent upon the response of my white cells and on occasions I'd get a reduced dose of 5mg, at other times I'd get no treatment in order to allow my healthy cells to recover, most importantly, this was all explained to me. Failure to consider my white cell count and just give the treatment would suppress my white cell population and importantly my ability to fight infection and therefore, any opportunistic infection could be a life threatening infection. In many respects, the drug, Vinblastine, a type of Vinca Alkaloid does not normally have such a damaging effect on the white cells and that is one of the reasons that the drug is used. However, I'd already had a significant amount of chemotherapy previously which had not seen my bone marrow recover completely. (The bone marrow is where our cells, of all descriptions, are made. It is also the target area for cytotoxic chemotherapy).

At my appointment on 9th June 1977, although there was no palpable disease (detectable on physical examination). I did have some problems with my arms specifically. I was experiencing pain in both arms and on examination, my reflexes were absent in the left arm and diminished in the right arm. In addition, I was having a strange toothache like attack from time to time. Question was, was this as result of the drug, known to cause peripheral neuropathy and jaw pain, or was it due to active disease? I got no indication as the answer of this dilemma, but equally, I did not ask the direct question either. The Vinblastine was continued at full dose, but the period between treatments was lengthened to three weeks.

Exactly three weeks later, I was experiencing pain and an absence of reflexes in my biceps, wrists and left triceps and in addition, my eyesight was slightly blurry. Dr. Atkinson assures me that this is probably a result of the medication and therefore, suggests that I have a break from treatment until these symptoms resolve. Furthermore, and most encouragingly, he states that there is no evidence of any disease, *"as far as he can tell"*. I am appreciative of his reassurance, however, there have been so many set backs that my mind races with the fear that the symptoms currently being manifested are due to the disease and my stomach reminds me that I am terrified of a return of the disease.

Fortunately for me and after a few weeks without treatment I returned to hospital for a check up and consideration of my future management. What a relief when Dr. Atkinson tells me that my bloods are fine and after a physical examination there are no lymph nodes to be detected. The symptoms previously reported have now subsided and I am convinced that perhaps this really was due to the chemotherapy. In fact, Dr. Atkinson decides that more of the Vinblastine injections are warranted.

Of course, I had still not been privy to the knowledge that this treatment was designed at being palliative in nature and despite the fact that I have the utmost of respect for the doctors and nurses who got me through the most difficult time of my life, who nursed and cajoled me through the real possibility of an early death, I am still to this day bewildered that there was so much collusion in respect to what was my illness, my treatment, my future. But, I now have to accept that as a matter of fact, to do otherwise would cause me to self-destruct. Today, the health care system has thankfully moved on since those times and patients and carers should be empowered to be part of the decision making process alongside the health care professional. Individuals with a potential cancer diagnosis need and demand as much information as they themselves can cope with. Therefore, information requirements must be patient driven.

Chapter Seven

Those five words were crystal clear and I hear them many times in my head, even today and to my dying day, I will not forget that particular moment more than any other during my traumatic experience.

Wind Of Change

During July 1977, I had the pleasure and fortune to visit America and as I'd never been out of the country before I was filled with excitement and anticipation. As I had now spent so much time having treatment both as an inpatient, but also as an outpatient, I had little enthusiasm to socialise, perhaps occasionally, but more often than not, it would be the company of Hawkwind who were my almost constant companions, despite never having met them they were my best friends.

The side effects of treatment seemed to be ever present and quite simply, my get up and go had been corrupted by this dreadful chemotherapy, while I had little idea of when it might return, if at all.

Subsequently, I had managed to save a few pounds that would subsidise my American trip. During the planning stages of my trip, I eagerly scoured the press in the hope of catching a glimpse of any programme on the television relating to America as I'd hoped to see the real stateside. Turns out that what you see on TV is of little similarity to true life in the states. I had planned to spend four weeks in North Carolina with Aunty Mary and her family.

My travel companion would be my Aunty Kathleen. She had not been to America either and promised to look after me should there be any medical problems although I had not given the health issue a second thought. As far as I was concerned there would be no problems especially as I had fully discussed the trip to America with Dr. Atkinson and Dr. Bozzino and they felt that it would do me good. Dr. Atkinson had arranged the appropriate correspondence for me to take should there be any problems and which would alert the medical staff as to the treatment I had had. Giving this important document little thought I placed it in my suitcase ready to take.

The planning all completed, in late July 1977 we headed off to North Carolina with huge aspirations, but also cautious optimism. We headed down the motorway as we were scheduled to leave from Manchester ring-way airport. Arriving by car at the airport, I vividly remember being taken aback as we drove into the airport, a large jumbo jet appeared to hover above us, almost motionless as it came into land; I had simply not realized the size of these aeroplanes, wow, these mothers were big! I admit to a degree of anxiety at that specific moment in time and a slight uneasiness about flying. However, there was no time for nerves now, we needed to check in and no sooner had we done this that we made our way into the departure lounge and then subsequently onto the plane.

The whole experience was something special and to this day I still get a buzz out of flying. Touching down in New York I was very excited, even though we needed another flight from New York down to Greensboro, North Carolina. The hussle and bussle of New York City certainly did not impress me and I found it no different from any other cosmopolitan city really. However, flying down to Greensboro, the significant difference was noticed when we stepped off the plane and I recall taking a deep breath, only to be stunned by the humidity which caught the back of my throat. This was awesome and I was well impressed. Not long ago and my future was so unsure, yet here I was standing on the tarmac of Greensboro airport in North Carolina, a different world completely to the one I'd left behind.

We collected our bags and met Aunty Mary and Uncle Jerry outside of customs control. I have to admit to being somewhat overawed by the whole experience. Outside in the car park and the car that Uncle Jerry was driving was a Grand Prix, and as you would expect in America, it was huge, a true gas-guzzler. The ride from the airport took around 45 minutes although it only seemed a few moments since we'd gotten into the car. The drive from the airport had left me feeling like a VIP, but equally, I had noticed the extremes of wealth. On one hand there were these luxurious beautiful houses, many of them with swimming pools and yet, there were others that were little other than wooden huts, looking as if the slightest gust of wind would blow them over.

Arriving at Pine Knolls, the house overlooked a magnificent golf course, although such was the summer heat and humidity that the grass was completely scorched. The inside of the house was of course air-conditioned and very palatial. I was sleeping in the basement bedroom, something of a complete contrast as to what I'd left behind in England, yet despite the obvious wealth, I was more than content with our small council house back home, particularly as my illness had taught me that you should appreciate anything that you have. In the house I was greeted by some of my cousins and it felt that I had known them forever. Over tea, we talked and talked about many different subjects, not least my illness and after a while, I had decided to put on a pair of shorts and take a walk around the estate. I had only strolled a few hundred yards passed the tennis courts and I heard the distinct southern drawl of '*look at that pair of skinny milk bottles*'. Naturally they referred to my white legs, still recovering from the destructive measures of malignancy and chemotherapy and of course, they weren't to know that and I had a little smile to myself.

Four glorious weeks in America was highlighted by a trip to the Great Smokey Mountains and then into Ooconaluftee Village, the Cherokee Indian Reservation, and the pinnacle of the visit. Pulling up in one of the car parks we were greeted by an artificial Indian made up especially for the tourist, he immediately stretched out his sun-baked hand waiting for the dollar bills that would allow us to take his photograph. Although there was lots of authenticity, there was also an awful lot of tourist junk. Anyhow, I bought some historical books and probably little else as I was completely overwhelmed by the surroundings and confused as to what I should and should not buy that when it was time to leave I had bought almost nothing.

The feeling of pride that these people (Indians) had despite their plight and despite the way that the American model had oppressed and undermined them was admirable. This truly was a humbling experience, a visit that lived up to all my expectation. These great people had almost been wiped out by the greed and avarice of unlawful settlers over many centuries and yet they had lost none of their resolve, something I associated with and my battle against cancer.

Driving from Ooconaluftee Village and the journey through the mountains was breathtaking and certainly something that mere words could not do justice too, in a small clearing we stopped the car and found a small gurgling stream, while there I bent over and sipped the crystal clear virgin water of Ooconaluftee River. Back in the car and on the way down the winding road of the Smokey Mountains the heavens opened and like everything in America, it's done on a much larger scale, and the raindrops were the size of golf balls and gave a new meaning to the word torrential. I do believe that the entire experience had a significant impact on my health and certainly played a part in my recovery and the entire experience was so impressive that I promised to return the following year.

During my stay in Americas Deep South, I met some real nice people, extremely friendly and boy, did they know how to cook. That good old southern food is second to none as was the hospitality. We also did an awful lot of travelling and saw some beautiful places and I would recommend the area to anyone. My cousins Karen, David, Shelley, Scott and Charles helped make the holiday a memorable one. One night Charles and I visited a night club and as we went in everyone was taken by my English accent, especially a bunch of Hells Angels who looked quite fearsome but turned out to be big Hawkwind fans and very friendly. All the way to America to bump into Hawkwind fans, now that's impressive, now that's fate. And so we talked music, shared joint after joint and discussed the experience of Hawkwind live as most of them had not had the pleasure to witness the band at first hand, they were a great bunch of guys and had many questions about Hawkwind that I was only too pleased to answer.

There were many parties organised and indeed at one of these I met a young girl called Melissa. After chatting most of the night I walked her back to her car and gave her a long lingering kiss which seemed to last forever. We arranged to meet the next day and the next again, she was gorgeous and I thought I was in love and her image filled my thoughts for months after my return to England, stupidly though, I did not get her contact details before my return home. Naively, I thought I'd return to America the next year and she'd be there waiting for me, but of course that never happened.

During my stay in North Carolina, Uncle Jerry and Aunty Mary took us all over that fantastic state. We had a great time, met some wonderful people, saw some spectacular sights and for me at least it was a complete escape from what I had endured the previous couple of years and it proved to be more than therapeutic.

Only days after my return from the states, 28th August, 1977 I was apprehensive of the need to visit the hospital for my requisite appointment, despite feeling so very well, in fact, I felt better than I had for many many months, but would I feel as well when I came out of the consultation? My reflexes were still not what they should be although in all honesty I had not realised any deficit and I had no specific symptoms. I waltzed into the consulting room and took my place on the examination couch, suddenly the butterflies were evident as Dr. Atkinson strolled in, his usual smile stretched across his face he asked how the holiday had gone and naturally, I was only too pleased to tell him. Like Dr. Bozzino, Dr. Atkinson would allow as much time as was required for me, this was important and didn't go unrecognised.

It was now over five weeks since my last injection and Dr. Atkinson was keen to continue with this treatment. My imminent question was when would they stop? The proposal was that a further six injections should be given at two weekly intervals. This I could accept for two reasons. The first was that the side effects were negligible from this chemotherapy and secondly, more importantly, Hawkwind were once again on the road and heading to Newcastle in September. Make no mistake about it; I'd be first in the queue while on this occasion I'd take my sister, Allyson with me. Now Allyson was usually into David Cassidy and other teenybopper music and therefore, I was dubious as to her reaction to Hawkwind but she new my passion for the band and was keen to accompany me. After the concert she was as enthusiastic as I, although her interest was not sustained, but most importantly she had enjoyed the night of live space rock and it gave me great pleasure to take her along to see such an important event.

I'd come this far now that it would have been foolish to stop treatment against the medical advice; what's more, I had endured chemotherapy so horribly worse than this, that any argument I had against this particular treatment really wouldn't be a strong one. I reluctantly agreed with Dr. Atkinson's opinion of more chemo, simply because I really did have faith in his clinical judgement as I did with Dr. Bozzino.

On completion of the Vinblastine injections, Dr. Atkinson explained that there would be a need to have me admitted to Newcastle for in depth investigations which would be required to determine whether there was any disease still in evidence. Unless there were palpable lymph nodes to feel or an abnormal blood count, there was no way to ensure that the treatment had been successful. Therefore, I agreed to his request but emphasized that I could not be in hospital on 20th September or the 5th October. On those dates I had two significant and most important appointments, the first at the City Hall in Newcastle and then followed by another journey to London, this time onto the Hammersmith Odeon to see a certain band called Hawkwind. There was no doubt that my inspirational band had kept me going through so many emotional and difficult tribulations that I would travel anywhere to see them. More importantly, I had missed the Hammersmith Odeon gig the year before; it would be a brave man who tried to stop me now.

True to his word I was admitted to Newcastle General Hospital at the end of November 1977 for a week of invasive tests and investigations which would make or break my future, tests which may make or break my spirit once and for all. Alighting from the lift on ward 38 I noticed plenty of familiar faces from a nursing perspective but, no Tom or anyone else that I recognised. In fact the ward was quite quiet and I ended up getting a cubicle, now this was preferential treatment. That same day I had a bone scan and also a series of X-Rays. Of course, on more than one occasion blood was removed from my accommodating veins.

Now, what I had done was make my own way up to Newcastle about a thirty minute drive from South Shields in my little car, a white Hillman

Imp and I had parked it just outside of the hospital and although ward 38 was on the fifth floor, I could see the car from the toilet window, a small point worth remembering.

The following day I was scheduled for a lymphangiogram investigation. This assessment of my lymphatic system was undertaken at a time prior to the availability of CT scans. Subsequently, I was taken into the treatment room and made comfortable on the examination couch, after which my feet were cleaned with antiseptic solution, then, local anaesthetic (lignocaine) was injected between my first two toes and boy did that stuff sting when it went in. On the top of each foot an incision approximately an inch in length was made, from this the lymphatic channel could be accessed and a special coloured solution was infused over a two-hour period. The infusion was a special type of blue dye that would circulate the lymph system and allow a series of X-Rays to highlight this part of my anatomy and from this an assessment could be made regarding any residual cancer being present. In addition, the blue dye turned not only my urine blue, but also gave my skin a blue tinge. Following the procedure, my feet were stitched and I was expected to remain in a wheelchair for at least twenty-four hours.

Anyhow, following the lymphiangogram investigation and in my infinite wisdom I decided to go down and check the car and ensure it was ok and that the battery wasn't flat. Therefore, I steered my wheelchair into the lift and down to the ground floor, in a few moments I was now out into the open air. The car park was slightly downhill; actually it was more down hill than I thought. Initially, it wasn't too hard to control the wheelchair, but as the chair gathered more and more momentum I lost control and how I didn't tip completely out of the contraption is something I'll never understand. So here I am rolling down the hill and directly towards my little car and as I was unable to stop the chair I crashed into the side of my little white car!

Now, my biggest concern was not for my feet, not for my car and certainly not for the wheelchair, I was more concerned that someone would be looking out of a window and would have seen my fiasco. All three were satisfactory and only my pride was dented. I slowly made my way back up to the entrance of the hospital, into the lift and back onto the ward, paranoid that someone must have seen the mishap. No one ever admitted to seeing me but I'm still not certain that some of the staff had not seen the spectacle and had a dammed good laugh, if I'd seen such an event, then I would certainly have busted a gut laughing.

After all of the requested tests I was discharged home, although it would be another week before the entire test results had been collated and sent to Dr. Atkinson. It was going to be a long week, a very long week, I would soon realise just how long seven days would feel. Despite being at work during the day, my mind was filled with the potential test results, they must be positive as I felt so well. The days seemed to linger and doubt almost inevitably crept into my thoughts, particularly as so many times in the past, the cancer came sweeping back to invade my fragile system. So, there were certainly times when I was the eternal pessimist. Dr. Atkinson knew what this meant to me and therefore, if the results proved positive and in my favour, then surely he would have been in touch to put me out of my misery. As I hadn't heard from him I began convincing myself that it must therefore be bad news and I convinced myself that the tests showed the presence of cancer and that more chemotherapy would be required. Night time was the worst; there was no settling, as my mind required the answers to those fundamental tests. I tossed and turned on many a night leading up to the hospital visit when the results would be disclosed. Unable to sleep, I'd get up and sit reading magazines and listening to the good old faithful, Hawkwind. My mind unable to focus for more than a few seconds on any reading I'd eventually drop off to sleep sitting in the chair, awaking in the early hours un-refreshed and irritable.

The last few days leading up to the Thursday appointment, my mind was filled with trepidation and what the results would show. If it was bad news, was I ready for more treatment? Could I take any more treatment? Would more treatment be offered, even if it were bad news? After all, I'd relapsed now four times in the face of active chemotherapy and indeed, radiotherapy.

Thursday arrived and alone by choice, I headed off to hospital anxious as never before and as always, I went straight to the blood room to have the usual blood count done. Significantly, the blood room was directly up the corridor from where the clinic was held and as I walked sluggishly along the corridor from the blood room I was alarmed to see Dr. Atkinson standing in the doorway and although I was some thirty feet away from him, he suddenly and unexpectedly threw his arms in the air and shouted at me *'you're all clear, bloody clear'*. Those five words were crystal clear and I hear them many times in my head even today. Was this a dream, did I hear correctly, had it all been a dream? No, despite this fantastic news, I was somewhat bemused as to how I should react to this million pound award. As I drew up close to Dr. Atkinson he took my hand and firmly shook it with true commitment and graciousness, I began to fill up with emotion, not knowing what to say to my friend who had given me such an astonishing gift. To my dying day, I will not forget that particular moment more than any other during my traumatic experience.

This was quite amazing, all that aggressive and debilitating chemo-therapy, relapse after relapse after relapse, the onslaught of Yuletide radio-therapy and even a further relapse. Then followed treatment with a drug given not with the intention to cure, but merely to control specific symp-toms, ironically, this was the drug that would cure my cancer. That's it! Eventually, the treatment is finished; it's time to move on and naturally, regular reviews would be required although I knew deep down that I was far from out of the woods. Let's not tempt fate by being overtly optimistic, but even so, I went home on an artificial high, drunk on euphoria, desper-ate to share my news with the world.

Was this possible? The treatment was finished, was I in the clear, well, certainly for now, yes. But, what of the future? That was a little uncertain. It had been a long, hard and emotional battle; the disease and ultimately the treatment had taken hold of me and attacked me from every conceiv-able angle, not one solitary part of my body was spared the vanquish of the disease, my mind included. My adolescence had been taken away and my sanity stretched to the limit. Even my testicles had shrunk as a conse-quence of the drugs I'd received and my mortality had visited the edge of time more than once, not to mention the savage side effects which pushed my physical being onto an undiscovered plane. However, strangely, I felt good about the entire experience, it had taken so much from me, but, it had given me so much more. An appreciation of life, a focus previously unknown and a promise to myself to live life to the full taking each and every day as it came, life is to short to do anything else.

Sadly and regrettably I had refused to have any photographs taken during the entire cancer journey as I did not want any reminder of the experience, even though my mind was permanently and painfully full of the thoughts I desperately wanted to discard, but couldn't.

Over the following twelve months I would continue to attend the diagnostic centre for check ups, initially this was monthly, but then, three monthly and almost expectedly, prior to each visit I would be anxious about the outcome and in these bizarre situations it was amazing the way the mind would play such outrageous games. Will they tell me the cancer is back? Will I get confirmation that I'm still clear? Will they not know and I'll need more tests? Of course, at each visit I would get the all important ratification that my body was free of any signs of cancer and between visits I would once again see my beloved Hawkwind and I would extract the usual well being, inspiration and positive vibes that they had given me during my difficult treatment. Not surprisingly, my mind would begin to fill with those fears and concerns weeks prior to each visit for each check-up and no matter how well I felt. Deep down I knew how well I felt yet I simply could not prevent these unwanted and demanding questions entering my mind.

Towards the end of 1978 I did return to America, this time I visited Tennessee as Aunty Mary and Uncle Jerry had moved. On this occasion, I would stay for ten weeks taking in many more sights, but not forgetting a return visit to Ooconaluftee Village in the Smokey Mountains and a visit to the mystical Cherokee Indians. Naturally, I never did see Melissa again but hey, there were plenty more girls to have fun with. There was even a time when I thought I would emigrate to America and start from scratch. Thinking logically of course I would never get insurance, let alone any worthwhile work, so that idea was soon history. Many years in the future I would visit many of the other states in America and it remains a favourite place to visit and explore.

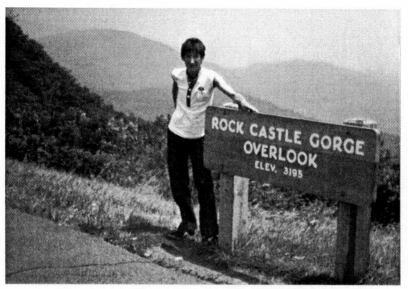

At last, chemotherapy behind me. But still underweight

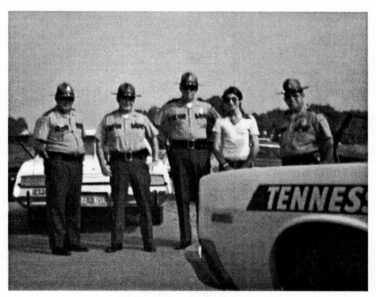

Outnumbered in Tennessee

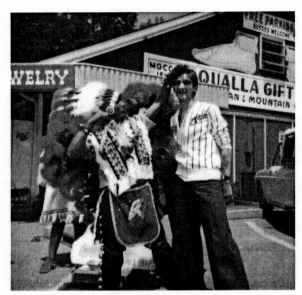

Black Elk speaks

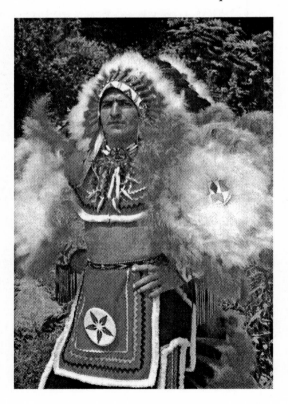

*Chief Henry of the
Cherokee Nation*

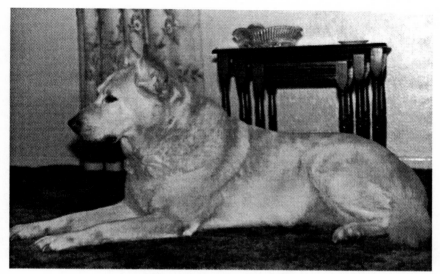

Sheba, my protector and friend

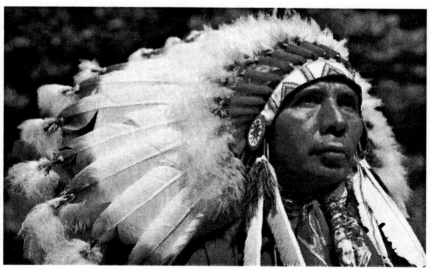

Cherokee Indian Chief

Chapter Eight

In the first instance of marriage, the shuddering reality of a cancer diagnosis would soon become evident and prove that the final whistle of a cancer diagnosis never blows.

Rocky Paths

As illness had played such a significant part of my life and had at times been an all consuming event, I had missed out on so much that others had taken for granted and of course not forgetting, when I did have the opportunity to get out and about, I preferred to travel the land and see Hawkwind at every opportunity and importantly, I had no regrets regarding this. Hawkwind had supported me, kept me focussed at the most difficult times throughout my youth and yet, much of my teenage years had been ruthlessly taken from me without my consent, adolescence had not been normal for me, how could you call a cancer affliction normal? Still, I could not allow it to continue and it was time to move forward.

As we moved towards the end of the seventies many of my friends began to make plans to marry, Colin, Dave, Alan, Keith, and both Mickey's had tied the proverbial knot, and yet, I could count on one hand the girlfriends that I'd had, all prior to my illness. Sadly, and all for the wrong reasons I felt the urge to settle down, to normalise life, and so it proved to be the wrong decision.

In 1979 I met my first wife and naturally in hindsight it was easy to see that this would never work out and I take full responsibility for that, a knee jerk reaction on my part to be the same as everyone else and be recognised as normal. For so long, I had not been able to do the things that everyone else had been able to do due to the restriction placed on me by cancer and its subsequent demands. Not only did I miss so much of my adolescence, I missed the journey of discovery that is known as the opposite sex. However, in retrospect and in the fullness of time, my newfound girlfriend would prove to be a very jealous and bitter woman, an only child, previously spoilt by ageing parents. But that said, in all marriages, there are always faults on both sides and this would prove to be no exception. In my own defence and hand on heart, never in eighteen years of marriage did I ever give her any reason to be jealous, yet later down the years, I would be accused of having affairs with nurses, my best friend's wife and even other men, not one of these accusations had any credence or substance. But importantly, this is not the time to dwell on past mistakes.

After a brief courtship, less than twelve months in fact, we decided to get married later in 1980. This was a time that was supposed to be the start of the rest of my life, the building blocks of the future. Moreover, this was supposed to be a time that couples look forward to and it was intended to be a moment in time when I was attempting to put the realms of cancer behind me, to move my life forward as everyone else had done. That would prove more difficult than I had ever thought and of course, not the ideal foundation of a marriage, in that regard, I take the blame for its ultimate failure.

Week's prior to the intended wedding; Hawkwind had released a fantastic new studio album, Levitation. On a number of nights, I confined myself to my bedroom and blasted out this outstanding album and contemplated my future, was I doing the correct thing? So many questions running around my mind but no answers were forthcoming and in many respects, I was not strong enough to suggest to myself that this marriage was not the right move.

Even the night before the wedding, a blazing row erupted between my future spouse and I and words were once again exchanged that could have and should have stopped the actual ceremony taking place. It's an amazing little phrase, what if? Unfortunately, that is now part of history and part of what ultimately became part of my own fate. More importantly, it is not my intention to blame an ex-wife for the ineptitude of a failed marriage. It takes two to succeed and also two to fail. So let's just leave it at that.

In the first instance of marriage, the shuddering reality of a cancer diagnosis would soon become evident and prove that the final whistle of a cancer diagnosis never blows. We had decided that a mortgage would be the first rung on the ladder of life. Sadly, that would never be realized until many years in the future, as the first visit to the estate agent would be the last. The privilege of having been bestowed a cancer diagnosis means that a mortgage is not something that is readily forthcoming, in fact, the estate agent, without compassion, declares we won't be able to offer you a mortgage, neither will anyone else. Very soon after that misfortune, I discovered that there would always be someone prepared to take advantage of the fact that my personal history included being plagued by the blight that is cancer. Why? Well, when it comes to taking out life insurance, those friendly mutual societies had already decided that cancer patient's are a huge risk and, because of that risk then you must pay the premium, which means you pay twice the normal premium and not just that, the policy has specific restrictions. Sadly, in the game that is life, as a cancer patient, even one that is cured, you just cannot win and I felt exploited.

Regardless of the early marital obstacles, things were ok for a short while until talk came around to starting a family. Naturally, that was something both of us wanted. Life just isn't the same without children and we both agreed that at least two children would be ideal. Unfortunately, nothing seemed to be happening, month on month and although it was still early days, something prompted us to seek help from the family doctor. Was it her or was it me who had a problem? Or, was it that we simply had not given it enough time?

So, an appointment was made and off we went to see our family doctor, the doctor appeared rather nervous when confronted as to why we had not gotten pregnant. A nice guy, his discomfort obvious as he squirmed in his seat and informed us that in all probability, we would not be getting pregnant as the type of drugs (chemotherapy) that I had received some years earlier would ensure that sterility was assured. I was stunned, speechless, no one had ever approached this scenario, and I could not recall any health care professional even intimating that this might be a problem. Now I felt gutted, tearful and also very angry. What an impressive encore following on from the massive stage performance that is cancer.

Cancer doesn't just stop influencing your life once treatment has been completed, it was surely influencing mine now and believe me I was angered. I think on reflection I was angered more by the medical fraternity than the actual disease. The disease itself could have quite literally taken my life, but, instead I had survived and had developed a healthy respect for this most unforgiving of debilitating conditions. No, the doctors must have known that this would be the result or perhaps the truth is that they didn't expect me to survive. In addition, I did feel as though I had misled my wife, although not intentionally. She was now in a position where she was struggling to come to terms with this unfortunate situation, as we both were. Yes, I was clear of the dreaded disease and of course I was grateful for that, but the bitter taste that it had left behind took away my anticipation and determination to be a parent.

A couple of weeks later and we decided that we would not be beaten. The answer, adoption! Unfortunately, it was not to be that easy, following enquiries to Barnadoes, Durham Dioceses and a handful of other well-established adoption agencies we were declined without hesitation or explanation. Even the local social services decided that because of my background of cancer, and then we were not fit to be considered to be prospective adoptive parents. A Further appointment with our doctor and we where referred to a specialist in fertility treatment, AID (artificial insemination by donor) was the option we chose in an attempt to be parents. Sadly, the Consultant was based in Sheffield; however, if it meant a child, then the journey would be comfortably worthwhile, as would the wait. The current waiting list was around ten months.

Ironically, the fostering and adoption officer at the local social services left to have a baby and the incoming officer, Maggie had apparently been reviewing all of the old files and had discovered our file and was bemused as to why we had not been considered for at the very least, fostering. Maggie contacted us and asked if she could come and visit. Not only was this the start of a professional relationship it was also the beginning of a great friendship too. Maggie explained that there was no reason why we could not, in the first instance foster children with a view to long term fostering and subsequently and hopefully, adoption. Maggie agreed after that first meeting to put the wheels in motion. References and police checks were an integral part of this system.

In less than six months, interview after interview, we went before a matching panel with a view to be considered for a fostering position with a child currently in short term placement, her name was Donna. The matching went well as did the interrogation, sorry, the final social services interview.

You know, it seems ironic that social services go to so much bother checking out prospective parents and yet seem to have little power in stopping biological parents breeding like the proverbial rabbits and subsequently treating children like animals. We've all read about these cases in the press and yes, I was bitter toward those parents who apparently had little interest or dedication when it came to the security and well being of innocent children, parents who regularly neglected their offspring. I was certainly frustrated and angry at the hidden destruction that cancer had had on my future. Naturally, the police and character checks made prior to allowing couples to adopt or even foster children are essential and I had no argument with that process.

Anyhow, Maggie explained that Donna was in need of some long-term stability and she felt that we were the people to offer it. Trepidation is an understatement regarding the couple of hours leading up to our rendezvous with Donna. We had met the foster parents of Donna at a separate meeting along with Maggie; however, when we eventually got to meet Donna for the first time, we travelled there alone and although only a ten minute drive from our home, it seemed to take forever to get there such was the apprehension and fear, perhaps Donna would not take to us, perhaps she would break out into uncontrollable tears at the site of us. At the short-term foster parents we were ushered into their front room and the mum brought Donna downstairs. What a little picture, Donna was a two year old with large brown hypnotic eyes but no smile to offer. She had mousy, shoulder length hair that was allowed to just hang and the clothes that she wore were nothing special, unlike the clothes worn by the short term foster parents natural children. More importantly, she would come nowhere near me. Still, this was the first visit. An hour later, we left and agreed to visit again the following evening. At this next visit, Donna almost forgot her previous fear and immediately brought me one of her toys; she tilted her head and offered to me the slightest hint of a smile. That smile, or part of a smile, meant a great deal for me, it meant acceptance after such a short period of time. Donna had had so many moves in her short life that she actually was too friendly towards strangers. She had sadly, known so many different homes that I'm sure, even though she was only two years of age, probably realised that another was imminent.

It had been agreed that the sooner Donna moved in with us then the sooner we could try and establish some rapport with her. On Saturday we headed over to Washington to collect Donna and I shall never forget leaving that house with Donna and her sole possessions, all crammed into a brown paper carrier bag. It wasn't hard to deduce why the short term foster parents took Donna and others like her, the financial reward!

It was a beautiful summer Saturday afternoon and no sooner did we get home than we thought that the more we can do to keep Donna occupied the better, this was undoubtedly going to be a very difficult time for Donna and her re-adjustment, still, she would be the focus of our attention. Lunch was first on the agenda, followed by chocolate pudding. Now every parent must have a picture of one of his or her children having just devoured some type of messy food. This was no exception and Donna was covered from one end of her infectious smile to the other and that made a great photograph. Donna enjoyed the afternoon and during the early evening she fell asleep on the couch. Therefore, it was important to start and get Donna used to a routine, so, off to bed. However, once washed and into bed, it was heartbreaking that Saturday night when Donna was placed into her new bed, her inconsolable tears were, from that time onwards, indelibly imprinted on my mind. The same pattern was repeated for at least a week until she eventually settled. From a parents point of view, things went from strength to strength as far as Donna was concerned and very quickly I new deep down that I loved her as only a father can.

Days later and a letter arrived on the mat inviting us down to Sheffield for the fertility appointment. Donna, although only a few weeks into her stay, was now an important part of our family and therefore, she would come along with us. The meeting with the condescending Consultant was both short and to the point. After a brief interview, which saw my wife and I explaining who Donna was, he astounded us with his decision in respect to considering us for artificial insemination. There was no hope, his view was that he did not advocate single parent families and flatly refused to consider us for AID. This of course, was a direct reference to my personal history, a history of cancer. The impact of cancer can be so devastating, even when all of the treatment is complete and you are trying to establish yourself back into society, it has a way of rearing its ugly head to kick you in the teeth. In fact, that's not strictly true; it demonstrated the ignorance and lack of compassion of certain individuals, even those in the so-called caring profession. I was so taken aback that I could not wait to get out of there and head back up the motorway to civilisation. How could a Consultant be so insensitive and without empathy? If that was his opinion, then fine, but surely as an intelligent man he should have learned a degree of diplomacy.

Life was now about enjoying Donna and the pleasure she could bring. Sadly, she was rather slow in her psychological development, put down to all of the moves she had had in her short life according to the health visitor. This lack of developmental progress was the last thing that concerned me as Donna was an absolute joy and brought family fulfilment, at least in those early years.

It seemed that life was at last becoming normal; I was doing what was expected, enjoying family life. Things just don't have the ability to go that smoothly for too long in my experience and so it proved. I was devastated and concerned in 1984 when I was again taken poorly. Night sweats and a general deterioration in my health and I found myself confined to bed and had been for around seven days. The emergency on call doctor was summoned as I was now getting worse and drifting in and out of consciousness and after his examination, he rang for an ambulance and had me admitted directly to Sunderland Royal Hospital late that night.

The following days were something of a blur, but test followed test, something I was familiar with and although the suspicion was malignancy it proved to be a significant viral infection. The worst of the tests was a lumbar puncture, something new to me but not something that I would be in a hurry to have repeated. The important fact is that it clearly diagnosed a viral the infection and the appropriate treatment was initiated. Five days later and I'm on my way home to continue the rest of my life. The huge problem with a cancer diagnosis is that the affected individual makes an assumption that any cough, cold or other health problem must be a recurrence of the dreaded disease. Now I do not believe that this is a paranoid tendency, it is an understandable reflex, a fear that cancer was again about to dominate my life and threaten my mortality. But then thinking about it laterally, just because you've had cancer, doesn't mean that you will not get anything else, of course you can and will, whether its a simple cold to general aches and pains, it's simply about trying to rationalise and put everything into perspective.

As I have discussed previously, the diagnosis of cancer doesn't just stop exerting its effects on an individual simply because the treatment has finished, even when a cure has been discussed and the chemotherapy is long finished. Remember, earlier I discussed about the strange effects of the Vincristine as it was being administered during the time when I was having chemotherapy, the experience of a weird taste and inexplicable sense of smell as a result of this particular drug and, because of this weird and nauseating sensation, I would drink orange during its administration to try and diminish its effect. Well, some five years from completing my own cytotoxic chemotherapy and which had proved a difficult time to say the least, I happened to be walking along a country path one day during the summer when the most nauseating smell filled my nostrils, the smell of Vincristine, making me feel physically sick. But, what was this unusual phenomenon and where was it coming from? It turned out that the smell came from a common countryside weed, called Rosebay Willow, also known as bombweed or fireweed and unfortunately, it litters the English countryside. Sadly for me, the smell that it delivered was a smell exactly like the drug that was administered into my fragile veins so long ago and strangely, I associated the smell with the unique taste of that drug, Vincristine. It was during this summer amble that my inner senses were confused by this phenomenon, my psyche aggravated, my fears and darkest thoughts rekindled. That was a bewilderment that I had not expected and the smell immediately provoked a physical sensation of nausea and the dreaded memory of what it was like to have chemotherapy. Even today, I will go out of my way to avoid any contact or proximity with fireweed such is the strong association it has with the treatment I received. It's a strange old world.

Chapter Nine

At this moment in time with the impending doom we had to try and think laterally. Our little girl had been passed from pillar to post throughout her brief existence, she had known no continuity until now and yet according to the doctors she was dying.

Lord Of Light

It was now 1985; some year and a half since Donna became an invaluable member of the family and things were going as they should, or so I thought. It was a Saturday morning and the usual routine would be followed, I'd get up with Donna and make the breakfast, then get dressed and take a ride into town. This particular morning I was washing Donna when I discovered a lump the size of a walnut on her left elbow. Strange, I could not remember that being there the previous week I thought to myself. Naturally concerned, I hurriedly got myself and then Donna dressed and headed straight down to the doctors. *"Nothing to worry about, a simple infection in her arm is all that this is and antibiotics will sort it out"*, was his response. Donna was otherwise well and therefore, I had no reason to doubt him and so I left the surgery and collected the antibiotics and then headed off home.

Seven days later, the lump was still there, no bigger and yet no smaller and so, back to the doctors again. *"Different antibiotics are needed, the infection hasn't responded to the previous antibiotics"* according to the doctor as he insisted this remained a simple infection, demonstrated by the fact that after he had examined Donna and there was now a lump in her neck too, clear evidence in his view that this was an infection. Despite being dubious regarding his diagnosis, I thought to myself, he is the doctor after all and we had never had any problems with him previously and so I again, accepted his explanation and headed off to the chemist to arrange for the next antibiotics. Less than a week later there was absolutely no change. This time, I was not messing about and I took Donna straight to the Accident and Emergency department to see a Paediatrician, but even there, when I tried to express my concerns to the on call doctor, he was quite dismissive of my concerns. As if to appease my nagging, a blood test was taken and showed a marginal anaemia and an elevation of her white cell count which potentially would go hand in hand with an infection, however, as far as the doctor was concerned this was nothing to be concerned about and we were asked to make an appointment for the Monday on the children's ward in Sunderland Royal Hospital. Sounded to me as if the medical fraternity were closing ranks and not prepared to take my worries seriously. I new from my own experience of illness that an elevated white count can be seen in a number of infective states, but of course it could also be the first indication of something more sinister and therefore, I felt that at least, it warranted further investigation, particularly as Donna had already had had antibiotics for fourteen days without any response.

As requested, Donna attended the children's ward on Monday and had a variety of tests done during that week, including a biopsy of the lump on her arm that was causing so much of my concern but despite all of the investigations she ran around the ward like an Olympic athlete. The Consultant in his infinite wisdom decided that this was sufficient proof that Donna was a healthy fit youngster, strangely basing his diagnosis on this fact alone and subsequently Donna was discharged home with no specific medical condition being detected. Instead, the Consultant declared that she would be as right as rain in no time. Having no experience of health care other than my own illness, who were we to argue and therefore, we did exactly that, took her home expecting her to resume normal activity. If the Consultant felt there was little to be concerned about, then who were we to question that statement?

Later in the middle of the following week, I remember getting a phone call at work asking me to attend the hospital for the test results and I distinctly remember driving from Wallsend to Sunderland thinking it must be something serious. However, my thought was that this could be, perhaps diabetes, something of the nature that was relatively easy to treat;

never did I ever contemplate a malignancy. My wife was already at the hospital and we met in the corridor and hurried along to the ward where the ward sister greeted us as if she had been expecting us and directed us to two chairs placed uniformly outside of the Consultants office; we sat there like chastised schoolchildren awaiting the penance of the headmaster. During our wait, sitting there patiently, I vividly recall the Consultant saying to the ward Sister *"can you get some tea and stay in with me"*. Now overhearing this statement made me suspicious and my heart began to race, my mouth became dry as if stuffed full of cotton wool. I was concerned at what it was he was about to disclose. In we went and you could have knocked me over with a feather when the Consultant blurted out without any compassion *"what do you know about Lymphoma"*. A moments pause and I responded, *"are you saying Donna has a Lymphoma"*? His response was short and without feeling, *"Yes"*.

The sensation experienced at this devastating news left us both numb with shock, the turbulence of unrecognisable emotion was overwhelming, unexplainable and we were lost for words. How could life be so cruel? Surely, this cannot be happening but what angered me more than anything else was that we eventually, against all of the odds, we had the chance to share our lives with a bundle of joy, Donna, and yet she was facing the same life threatening scenario that I had done less than eight years earlier. Her future uncertain and she also faced that same debilitating treatment as I had, chemotherapy.

As the main centre for this condition was at Newcastle, we were told to report there the following morning to ward 16 South. But now back at home, who do we phone first, do we need to phone anyone just yet? Perhaps once we get to Newcastle, it'll prove to be something much more innocent. Was this grasping at straws, or was our hope justified? Remember, our family doctor told us that Donna had nothing more than an infection, the Consultant of Paediatrics told us that Donna was fine and too lively to be significantly poorly; perhaps he was right in that assumption after all. Donna, other than a few swollen lymph nodes, had no other symptoms and was indeed well. I suppose deep down my understanding of lymphoma told me that these were not innocent swellings, but, I did not want to believe that reality, I had to have my own hope.

We travelled to Newcastle the next morning reaching the Royal Victoria Infirmary shortly after the rush hour. We entered the hospital and made our way along what felt like an endless, green tiled Victorian corridor. Eventually arriving onto the oncology ward, were we greeted by the stench of antiseptic, a noticeable fear in the pit of my stomach. What's more, some children were lying on their beds; others were running around the ward, and many of whom had no hair, a permanent reminder as to why they were there. We were greeted by Liz, a young staff nurse who would become a good friend and confidante in addition to her nursing role during the forthcoming weeks and months. There was little doubt that the ward had a wonderful feeling to it, friendly and relaxed. Our first meeting with the Consultant outlined that unfortunately, a diagnosis for Donna was not as clear cut as we had been led to believe and she would require a number of other tests before confirmation of a diagnosis could be discussed and then the eventuality of treatment. However, one thing was certain, this was indeed a malignancy!

In those early days when blood was required and it was often daily, Donna simply offered her arm ready for the removal of the red substance, but as you would expect she quickly learned not to be so cooperative and over the coming days and weeks, there would be even more blood tests and occasionally swabs from here and from everywhere, scans and all kind of weird and wonderful investigations, so much so that Donna soon realised that she did not have to give her consent freely or to volunteer herself for tests that may appear to be quite innocuous on the surface, she very soon became suspicious of any member of staff who approached her and it became a battle, sometimes a battle of will and persuasion, but at other times it would be a physical battle to retrieve the required samples or to persuade Donna to leave the ward for another test.

We didn't know it at the time, but her cancer was in her bone marrow and the malignant cells where overcrowding this important space to such an extent that her healthy cells were unable to function or re-populate. Subsequently Donna would require blood and platelet transfusions regularly. One of the necessary tests was a repeated tissue biopsy, this time; the lymph node in Donna's neck was to be excised and sent for analysis and it needed to be done in theatre under a general anaesthetic.

Anyone who has escorted his or her child to theatre in readiness for an operation knows the fear and trepidation that runs through your system as you make the long journey down the busy corridor, the nurse running alongside the trolley trying her best to make Donna smile but failing miserably as she was well aware that something quite unpleasant was about to happen. And, when after a half marathon around the hospital you finally arrive at the theatre, it is now that the fear really kicks in, as I have already been unable to convince myself that she is in safe hands, the doubt overtakes and now controls my mind and all of its subsequent thoughts, what if! Silent screams trying to escape from inside my head, the pounding sound of each beat of my heart and the distinct dryness of my mouth as we try and put on a brave face for Donna as she holds on tightly to lolly lodle (her favourite doll). All too soon and it's time to let the anaesthetist do her job and a huge lump sticks in my throat, the sinking feeling that envelopes your persona when you're asked to return to the ward once the fairy wind (anaesthetic) has taken effect. Some hour and a half later and Donna returns safely to the ward and sleeps for the next hour, frustratingly, it was now time to play the waiting game, what exactly would the biopsy show?

Sometime later that week and Donna was about to start some chemotherapy as the diagnosis was made as non Hodgkin's lymphoma and required immediate treatment to prevent further advancement. The nightmare was about to commence, reliving and confronting my own fears in respect to chemotherapy, I knew exactly what this chemotherapy was capable of and I worried about Donna's ability to cope with this difficult treatment. My feelings of apprehension and trepidation were tempered by the fear and anxiety I had at having to watch Donna receive the chemotherapy drugs similar to what I'd received less than eight years previous. I struggled to accept the helplessness of seeing Donna undergo this chemotherapy and all of the memories it elicited for me. I felt completely useless, not being able to protect her or have the treatment in her place. Indeed, it was harder watching Donna receive the treatment than it was to experience a similar; painful voyage myself, and that was an almighty struggle, yet I would have happily accepted the entire nightmare again, if only it would have relieved the need for Donna to be put through that torment. In many respects however, Donna made life as easy as it could have been in that unenviable position, her infectious smile and lovable character, her innocence and trust in us as parents, and at times it felt as if Donna was supporting us rather than us her parents support her.

From the very moment that you take your first step on the road of cancer discovery, and then each and every day tends to merge into one, time is of little consequence anymore. The only thing that is of any importance is helping and supporting your child cope with what to them is an unknown commodity. You simply cannot explain to a child the full implications of a cancer diagnosis and particularly what the consequences of that diagnosis are. A return of that kaleidoscope of emotional turbulence was about to begin again, this time there was no question of not being strong, not being able to cope, I now had a parental obligation.

Many discussions took place with both the medical and nursing fraternity who had a wealth of experience in respect to supporting parent's address these extremely difficult situations. Many people may believe that the child has a right to know what's going on and attempts should be made to explain the meaning of a condition such as cancer. However, as many parents again will disagree and prefer to cushion their children from such exposure. Neither approach is correct, and yet, neither is wrong. The correct choice has to be the choice that is right for your child as you as a parent see it. Once you make that decision, no one can criticise it.

We decided that we would explain to Donna as best we could about this dreaded condition. The mutual support from other parents was incredible and it was a fact that you could not get through the nightmare without that support.

Donna was fitted with a special device that allowed the chemotherapy to be administered, blood to be taken and most importantly avoided the need for further needles to be stuck into her fragile veins. The device, known as a Hickman line has revolutionised modern day chemotherapy.

However, watching Donna having chemotherapy was far, far harder than having the treatment myself and this caused not only a reminder of my own trauma but also heartache as I felt helpless and unable to take away from Donna her pain and sickness as only a father should.

Donna soon lost her hair but in all honesty this really didn't bother her as much as it bothered us, primarily because ignorant people would stand and blatantly stare when Donna walked passed. Loosing her hair was also a constant reminder of the seriousness of her current disease, a life threatening disease.

She was supplied with a brown wig and at every opportunity she would wear this. However, when appropriate it would be whipped of in no time, often to the surprise of unsuspecting passers by. On one occasion between treatments, we had travelled to Blackpool, one of Donna's favourite destinations. During the visit Donna had asked for a candy floss and during the time she was eating this, the wind began to blow, causing her to get mouth fulls of hair. Therefore, she simply put one hand on the top of her head and with one quick tug and the wig was removed and with nonchalance she continued to devour the candy floss, the whole action took less than a couple of seconds. But, just as Donna had decided to take this action, a gentleman was walking close by and in doing so, he glanced to his side toward Donna and his bottom lip dropped almost to his feet as he observed Donna with the candy floss and her actions.

Hawkwind had been such an inspiration to me, could they help Donna? Well, in all honesty she didn't like the majority of their music. However, there were nights when Donna went to bed and I would lie at the bottom of her bed and play some of the more ambient Hawkwind tracks as she fell asleep, particularly Wind of Change.

Over the next couple of months and Donna got weaker and weaker and picked up one infection after another and required a number of hospital admissions. Indeed, she had her fourth birthday in hospital. Donna had some time off the treatment in an attempt that she could put on a little weight and generally get stronger; there was a need to weigh up the risk against the benefits of waiting to see if she improved. But after only two weeks, the team at Newcastle felt that it was important to recommence the chemotherapy as this cancer could not be left untreated. Sadly, following this treatment Donna appeared to suffer worse side effects than previously; Sickness and lethargy, no desire to eat and an inability to move out of her bed, she was deteriorating in front of our eyes.

There really is no known coping strategy for a parent when a child is struck by such an aggressive disease and therefore, I cannot even attempt to explain how we as parents got through that impossible situation. The real coping mechanism was Donna! Despite her illness and suffering, she made things so much easier for us. Even though she was so poorly, Donna was a rock and made us feel so very humble as did all of the kids who were also with her in that ward and suffering the same fate as her. As she was so stoical how on earth could we crumble in front of her? That said I would crumble once away from the confines of that hospital ward. Yet as a parent, nothing but nothing can prepare you for the assault and battery inflicted by an unseen condition and which affects every inch of your person. But somewhere inside you have just got to find the bravery and courage that's needed to support your child. Ultimately, you never loose sight of the determination, the focus that your child will get better. Yes, there are times when you doubt that, but even then, you must convince yourself that one day the nightmare will end, if you don't, you'll loose your mind totally.

22nd August 1985: Back in hospital at Newcastle for further treatment and things did not appear to going to plan. Donna was now so weak that I had to carry her from the car to the ward. The treatment itself was not having the desired effect against this vicious malignancy and therefore, further investigations where warranted, including a lumbar puncture, which would prove to be the crucial test.

Later in the evening, we were asked to go into the office with the Consultant. It was obvious by his demeanour that this was serious and not the news we wanted to hear. "*We do not think Donna can take any more chemotherapy*", asking for clarification of the implication of this and he said with heartfelt compassion "*I'm afraid there is no more we can do for Donna*", the very words that each and every parent fears, the words they never want to hear and I have no shame in admitting that I just broke down and cried, and cried and cried. My entire system tingling with shock, disbelief. Every conceivable emotion attacking my very psyche. Not knowing what to do, what to say, how to react, an impossible situation. Eventually, I recall sobbing the question to the Consultant that I really didn't want an answer too, "*how long does she have*"? Obviously that's a question that just cannot be answered with any accuracy. However, what he said hit me like brick wall in the face. "*She may go during the night, as she is so poorly at present*". The feeling this news elicits is without doubt, indescribable.

Apparently, this was not a non Hodgkin's lymphoma after all. The malignancy had mimicked this type of haematological cancer. In fact, they now thought that what she had was an extremely rare form of an adult cancer, called Chronic Myeloid Leukaemia. More importantly, there was no known treatment other than to keep her comfortable.

Donna was moved into a side room and we both stayed with her that night. Previously when she was in hospital we would take turns at staying. This proved to be the worst night of my entire life, up until this point in time anyhow! Donna was almost unresponsive in her consciousness requiring lots of medication to keep her comfortable, yet, despite our worst fears Donna did survive that night and the next and the next. However, the Consultant still felt that she would die and that we were living on borrowed time.

At this moment in time with impending doom we had to try and think laterally. Our little girl had been passed from pillar to post throughout her brief existence, known no consistency and yet according to the doctors she was dying. Our main concern then was that Donna had never been christened and despite the fact that the decision was not legally ours to make, we did, and Donna was christened in the chapel at the Royal Victoria Infirmary. The Charge Nurse, Steve, was her Godfather and her named nurse, Liz was made Godmother.

Afterwards and back on the ward, the staff had laid on a fantastic party for Donna and the other kids. That was a very special day indeed and although Donna lay on her bed throughout the proceedings as she was so very weak, she still managed to smile as the other kids and parents all made the effort to ensure that Donna was the centre of attention. There is little doubt that was an emotive and difficult afternoon, our thoughts unable to cope with the knowledge and persecution of the thought of losing our precious daughter. It remains the hardest concept to explain, you're told that your little innocent girl is going to die, yet, as you watch her from a distance it is impossible to believe, impossible to accept. How can you come to terms with this frightening dilemma, quite simply I do not believe you can? You can try and appease yourself that she will be going to a better place, perhaps. But irrespective, there is a huge void, a chasm waiting to engulf the rest of your life. Furthermore, you can try and put it out of your mind, but that quite honestly does not work, especially when Donna is there and making the whole process tolerable, in a strange sort of way and ironically, it seems that Donna actually supported us through that period. There really is no coping mechanism known to man that can prepare you for the death of a child.

The plan was to keep her comfortable with blood and platelet transfusions whenever they where required. This went on for almost ten days, after which time Donna was stronger than she had been in quite some weeks. Strong enough to consider home and so off we went on the understanding that we returned each day for monitoring. The uncontrollable need and necessity to remain positive day in and day out in the hope that Donna would remain well became an exhausting occupation. Talking with other parent's in the same predicament as us, they would profess to be positive of mind, and yet it was hard work convincing yourself to be positive. Within the seclusion and confines of your own home, time to reflect on the cancer that was engulfing your child, then that positivism would very often evaporate and seeds of doubt would often become overpowering. Soon we would receive the most unexpected news.

Interestingly, some months and completely unexpectedly Donna spoke about the night she nearly died. Donna could clearly recall floating above her bed and seeing both her mum and dad crying. Furthermore, Donna insists that she saw a tunnel with the most unusual pretty bright lights at the end. She then claimed that a voice told her, *"It is not your time, go back to your mam and dad"*. Now, I'm sure many will pour scorn on this so called out of body experience, this near death experience, call it what you will. But this was from the mouth of a 4 year old and without prompts.

Even today, we know so little about life itself, especially the mind. Of course stories such as these are not uncommon but do lead to compound what is a complex, but hugely interesting issue. Whether this is the mind playing games, our inner psyche or something else is not open for debate here, but whatever it is, it is a fascinating discussion for another day and importantly, this was the experience of Donna.

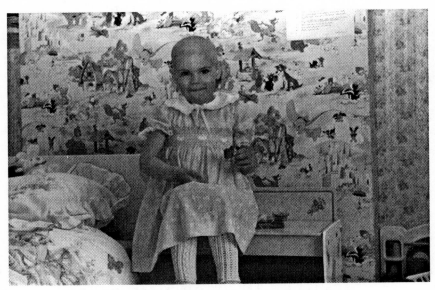

Donna, amazingly resolute despite the treatment

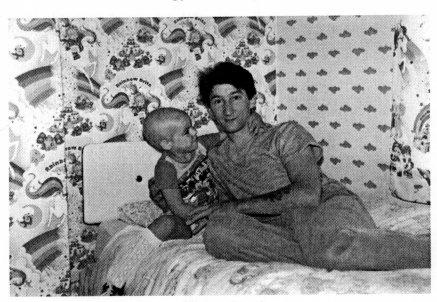

My best friend

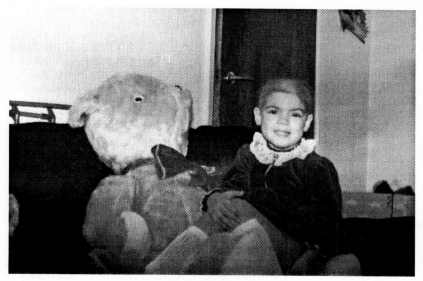

Donna and Bungle

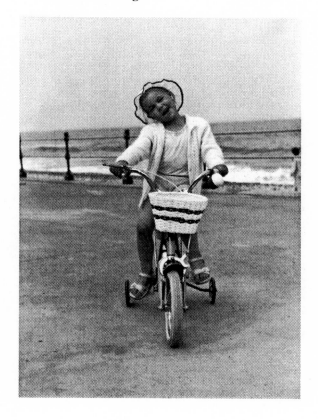

Life is for living

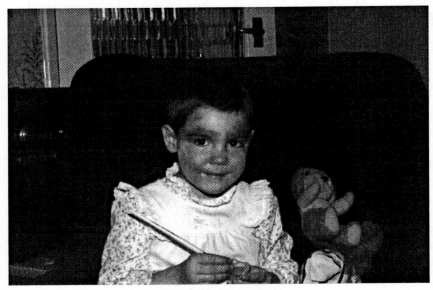

It's easy to find trouble

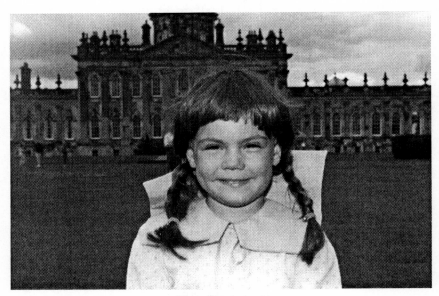

That famous wig

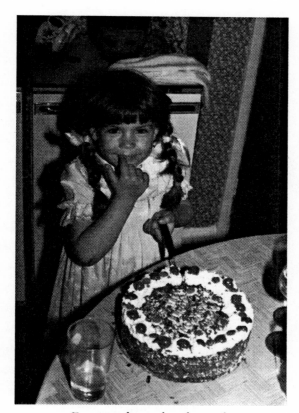

Everyone loves chocolate cake

Chapter Ten

Donna was all kitted out for her first day at school and she certainly looked a picture that inaugural day, her hair now just beginning to grow.

Quark, Strangeness, And Charm

B ack at home and one of the first things that I would arrange, in fact, something I should have done months earlier was the initiation of a daily dose of Ginseng for Donna. Was this grasping at straws? Probably yes, but who knows what significance it played in my recovery, perhaps none. But it could have been one of a handful of significant ingredients in my successful recovery from the cancer that had plagued my life. It was almost irrespective as to whether it had played any part in my recovery or not, what was important was that it certainly did no harm. And so, I went out and bought some Ginseng for Donna and she remained on the herb for many months, taking the elixir each morning without fail. Importantly, it could do no harm, although today it is now recognised that if you're taking this herb, you should ideally, take it for one month and then have a month's rest before starting again.

As Donna loved Blackpool, the plan was to spend all of the time we had left with her running back and forward to Blackpool although our first thought had been Disneyland in Florida, but we were advised against taking Donna out of the country such was the delicate state of her condition and the risk of infection or the potential for her health to rapidly decline. The dilemma was what should I do about work? I had been granted leave of absence from work due to Donna's deterioration, but what about long term? There was no way I could return to work with so much uncertainty surrounding Donna's very existence and therefore, I discussed this with the management and asked if I could be granted voluntary redundancy. Their response was tentatively yes, yet I suppose in many respects, this could have been seen as a knee jerk reaction by me. When Donna died, as predicted by the hospital, of course I would be bereft, but at some point I would need to return to work and this predicament just added to my confusion as to what the correct course of action was. Naturally, in situations such as this, logic does not come into the equation and I guess that's why management insisted on taking a little while to consider my request. Less than a week later, management asked me to call into work at my earliest opportunity to discuss the request of redundancy. They acknowledged the difficulty of the situation, offered to keep my job open indefinitely if I decided to continue to take leave of absence. However, my mind was made up; taking redundancy would give me the extra money I needed to do the things important to Donna and subsequently I took this option. This, as far as I was concerned, would allow me to do what Donna wanted and without the worry about finance. Once again, fate had played a significant role in my life.

Donna was a big wrestling fan. At the time Big Daddy (Shirley Crabtree) and Giant Haystacks were on the go. Naturally, like so many others, Donna was a huge Big Daddy fan. What a coincidence or was it fate? When we drove into Blackpool to see that there was a wrestling show playing that very night, including Big daddy, how fortuitous and therefore, once settled into the hotel my first job was to buy tickets for the show. I decided to try and locate Big Daddies manager, which I did without much trouble and I explained why, and how we were there and asked about the possibility of Donna meeting her hero. The manager said that would not be a problem and after the show, (incidentally, Big Daddy won his fight as expected) she asked us to head to the corner of the hall. Later that night and we did exactly as the manager had instructed; Big Daddy came out and invited us back to his changing room. He was absolutely superb, a true gentleman, more importantly, he was fantastic with Donna and spent a good while with her and he even told her that she was one of his heroes, what a moment of emotion. Quite an upsetting time, thinking that her life expectancy was limited, yet seeing her there with one of her heroes, it was all well worth it just to see her happy and content. Heading back to the hotel, that's all we heard about, Big Daddy, Big Daddy and more Big Daddy.

We returned to the North East the following day with Donna on a high and wearing her big daddy hat and scarf with pride. At hospital, everyone was told about her special friend, Big Daddy and the nurses listened intently to Donna's adventure and pride at meeting Big Daddy. After her examination and usual blood tests Donna was given a platelet transfusion, but, other than this, the Consultant was pleased with her. Therefore, one more day at home and then off to Blackpool again. It was almost as if Donna was a different girl compared to the young lady that night a few weeks ago. Occupying our minds with activities for Donna was not difficult and it was more than just a coping mechanism, even so, the night before every hospital visit was a major concern as to what would be said, what would be decided about her future?

As the weeks went by the visits to hospital became less frequent and each time the Consultant was amazed at Donna's blood profile and admitted to being completely baffled. That'll do for me and long may it continue was my silent thought, we didn't need explanations, as long as Donna was well. Discipline of any child is an extremely important parental responsibility and yet try and instil discipline when the child is expected to die; it is just an impossible task. Naturally, children soon realise that they can take advantage of a situation if they do not get instructed that they are doing wrong and that's exactly what happened with Donna. On the majority of occasions discipline was none existent, even if she misbehaved herself, so now was the time to put a halt to that mistake, even poorly children need to know wrong from the right, although it is a difficult transition once you have ignored for so long the misdemeanours.

Between trips to Blackpool Donna was sent to London by the charity, 'Dreams Come True'. But not just London, Donna had, for many years loved Jason Donovan and at this juncture in time he was playing the lead in Joseph and the Technicolor Dream Coat. Therefore, she got not just the opportunity to see the show; she also met Jason afterwards too.

The weeks, with dozens of trips to Blackpool, turned into months as Donna became physically stronger, stronger than she had ever been, although she remained susceptible to infection, her immune system still fragile from the consequences of chemotherapy. Yet, by their own admission, the Oncologist and Haematologist were both bemused at Donna's recovery. Neither able to confirm that they had any answers to this inexplicable recovery.

It was now that Donna had desires to go to school and although her friends had started some months earlier, we had been advised not to allow Donna to start as she remained immunocompromised (susceptible to infection). However, how on earth could we deny her this wish? Therefore, we discussed it with the hospital and they decided that it would probably be a good idea and one way of getting her back into some semblance of normality. And so we planned her attendance at school.

Donna was all kitted out for her first day at school and she certainly looked a picture that inaugural day, her hair now just beginning to grow. My greatest concern was the ridicule that she may have to endure due to the style of her hair or the fact that she was educationally slow. We all know how cruel kids can be, especially to each other and therefore I had great unease and a sense of nausea in the pit of my stomach as I led her away from home and it was a poignant journey that first trek to school.

In the playground, as the whistle blew, the lump in my throat refused to disappear as I tried in vain to put on a brave face as Donna turned to wave and smiled as she entered the doors for that first time. At least twice during that day I had deliberately walked passed the school in the desperate hope that I would catch sight of my vulnerable little girl. Anyhow, my fears proved unfounded as she came home that afternoon euphoric with stories of new found friends and the work that had been done.

Thankfully, the teachers had already had a discussion with Donna's classmates, explaining to some degree how poorly Donna had been and how she needed support from them all. During the first year, the majority of children did exactly that; support her, although there were exceptions.

School was good for Donna, at least for the initial year. After this time it was obvious that Donna was struggling with the work and this was becoming evident, particularly for the other children who at times would tease and taunt Donna. Children can be so cruel and in many respects that is almost understandable, but much to my disgust, one of the teachers was actually highlighting the fact that Donna was obviously different from the other kids and would emphasize this point by making Donna sit at the front of the class, on the floor and facing the blackboard. Donna was very upset about this and apparently, it had been going on for some time before one of the other children had mentioned this situation to us when she was at our house playing with Donna. Trust me, I was not about to let this one go; I demanded a meeting with both the head teacher and this individual to ask for some explanation, how on earth could this person call themselves a teacher? Furthermore, I demanded that it stop with immediate effect and although the head teacher was something of a wimp, his actions ensured that it stopped forthwith. It was obvious that something had to be done about this predicament and as parents; we would have been failing Donna had we not taken this action.

Now we know children can be very cruel. Donna's teacher's actions seemed to be an instruction to some of the children that Donna could be ridiculed. This bullying, teasing call it what you will was not going to go away. I felt that in view of what she had already gone through, then something must be done, on the other hand, the headmaster wanted Donna to continue as she was but, as parents we did not feel that this was acting in Donna's best interest and therefore, I contacted the educational psychology department for an official assessment and it proved to be the right move.

The assessment demonstrated that Donna had a mild deficit in her cognitive ability and had specific educational needs, a learning disability. Learning disabilities are seen in children who have epilepsy, kids who have had cancer in the first five years of life and also some adoption studies had demonstrated that learning disability is possible following adoption or fostering. Irrespective of the cause, this deficit could not be addressed by main stream education and subsequently she was placed in a school for children with both physical and mental difficulties.

At this establishment, Barbara Priestman School in Sunderland there was a great rapport between the children and most, although not all, of the teachers. Generally, Donna's time at this school was a happy one and significantly, it was a school that encouraged personal development of something inherent in each child. The philosophy was that each child had something they were good at. When questioned, Donna expressed a keen interest in swimming and a desire to improve the basic skills she already had. Her choice was brilliant and would certainly reap rewards for her in the not too distant future.

In her turmoil and understandable distress at the potential of losing Donna to the unpredictability that was a malignant disease. My then wife argued that we should investigate the opportunity of adopting another child. Now, this really did appeal to me, but, with absolute sincerity, I did not feel that this was the most opportune time, as there was still a huge uncertainty over Donna's future mortality. Yes, Donna at the time was well, but the hospital had warned us that she was far from securing a healthy future. In addition, she had recently been diagnosed with epilepsy that caused, on a bad day, hundreds of small seizures. However, my wife would absolutely amaze me with her rationale that if we adopted another child, it would be a replacement if Donna did die. Now I have to believe and see the best in people and perhaps this statement simply deflected her inability to believe Donna may still die from her cancer. But, this unbeliev-able statement flabbergasted me and in all honesty, I could have walked out, there and then. That however, was never an option, I am a believer in responsibility and as parents you have those obligations.

For weeks, there would be constant argument and disagreements over the merits of another child. Yes, I would and always did want more chil-dren; I simply did not feel that this was the most appropriate time. Despite the twisted and false allegations she would make in years to come about the issue, I feel that the protestations I made were correct at the time, they were never and are not a detraction from the subsequent events that followed. My main argument was the fact that Donna demanded so much focus of our attention and rightly so at that moment in time as her recovery contin-ued at a slow pace, such focus on her meant that another child, especially an adopted child, would not realise the attention they were entitled too.

Admittedly, I was weak when I succumbed to her constant pressure in respect to demanding another child. The now familiar adoption process was activated and eventually we got word that another child would be considered for placement with us. It would be a very similar process to what we had gone through with Donna and we would meet this little girl at the foster parent's home. On this occasion, it was evident that the foster parents were not doing this just for the financial reward. She was a well-presented young girl, aged two. She also appeared to be quite well adjusted with a happy demeanour.

Once introduced to her, I immediately forgot about my obstruction regarding further adoption. Importantly, the issue was never that I did not want another child and I never, ever, resented or regretted adopting another child. My argument was purely and simply the uncertainty that surrounded Donna and the possibility of further hospitalisation that would have interfered with the direct parenting and happiness that another adopted child was entitled to.

At two years of age, our new addition was a very intelligent red head who brought a new component of joy to the household and she was a support and companion for Donna. Donna equally, was a supportive and now proud sister. Her infectious smile would bring so much happiness and pride to my life, but, like all children, they would both cause upset at times, of course, as we all know, life as a parent will never be a bed of roses.

As a parent I always tried to instil into both Donna and her sister that they should remember one thing and this one thing has remained a key issue in my personal philosophy; No one person is any better than you are, but you are no better than anyone else. It is important in life to treat everyone in the same way that you expect to be treated yourself. Sadly, that is something some people find great difficulty achieving. It really does make life so much easier if we respect one another.

Following all of the treatment Donna had received, as I briefly mentioned, she developed epilepsy that by the admission of all of the experts would prove almost impossible to control. Indeed, for almost three years Donna was having hundreds of seizures on a daily basis. Just about all of the medication (anticonvulsants) available to medicine had failed to control the seizure activity. Remember, Donna had chosen to improve her swimming prowess, not something that usually goes hand in hand with epilepsy. However, contrary to popular belief, epileptics can swim, providing they have a recognised spotter on poolside, preferably someone who knows what to do in an emergency situation.

So it proved Donna would become more than just a prolific swimmer. The school did everything they could to encourage and promote Donna's skills. From my perspective, I joined Donna in a local swimming club to help develop her technique. To her credit, Donna worked exceptionally hard at her swimming and became quite adept. She comfortably achieved dozens of certificates and despite her cognitive deficits she could swim for miles and miles. 'If you think you can, you can. Always believe in yourself'.

Every year Donna's school would take part in a special schools event at Darlington's Dolphin Centre. This event was a variety of swimming events that for the successful individual could lead onto bigger and better things, even national events, including Special Olympics. At this event Donna had been entered into no fewer than six different races and here nerves were obvious, but I told her that this was all about concentrating on her ability and forgetting all about her disability. All of us are good at something, it's just a matter of finding exactly what that potential is and then honing it, if you think you can do it, you **can** do it! As the time drew closer and closer for her first competitive race, it was patently clear that Donna was physically shaking and doubt crept into her mind.

Donna stood on the side of the pool awaiting the starting gun, I marched up and down the poolside nervous and concerned, my stomach was in knots, and I hoped she'd remember everything about reacting to the gun and getting a good start. 'Take your marks' and then the gun goes, Donna flies through the air and streamlines into the water with a short lead. Halfway up the first length and all of a sudden Donna goes under the water and flounders. What seems like hours is only seconds and I'm flabbergasted that none of the life guards have gone in to rescue Donna as she was now having an epileptic seizure in the pool. Naturally, they had been informed prior to the event and had given her the go ahead to compete, so, as they hesitated and without a second thought, I ran along the poolside and fully clothed dove into the pool to rescue Donna. Meanwhile, at the same time, Donna's swimming instructor from school had realised too that nothing was being done and he was in there too. Donna was quickly pulled to the side and recovered from the incident. I will not highlight here what I said to the lifeguards, I'm sure you can guess.

It didn't end there either, what is so amazing that once recovered from the seizure, Donna insisted on continuing to compete in the remaining five races. However, even more amazing, she incredibly won three silvers and two gold medals that day. What an achievement! But that was just the beginning of her swimming adventure. On the bus home, the other school children congratulated Donna but really had a good laugh at Mr. Russell and myself and our premature swim.

Donna had now tasted competitive success and for the first time in her life realised that she could do something particularly well, she quickly learned that she excelled at this talent. And so, a new episode of adventure was about to take off. Donna was excited and was determined to train longer and harder to achieve her dream. With her allowance she would search out the very best equipment that afforded her the best opportunity of success and despite her educational deficit she would also become very knowledgeable in respect to qualifying times for different competitions and events.

Donna became a regular at the Darlington swimming event and won a bagful of medals over the years. On one occasion she was greeted by Tony Blair who had attended the gala to support the competitors. Donna was a very proud girl that day.

Donna became a regular in the local press and received much favourable recognition and awards for her swimming prowess. Naturally, when she came up against able bodied club swimmers she didn't fair as well, yet this never demoralised her. In fact, it probably proved to be a major motivation.

During 1995 Donna was invited to Rugby to try out for the England swimming team. The English Sports Association for People with Learning Disability was an excellent opportunity for Donna to receive top class instruction from first rate swimming instructors, but also the chance of representing her country. After her trial the head coach said she would like Donna to attend the next training day. From then on Donna was a regular in the English set up, although it would be a little while before she got into the actual team for an official event. The other individuals were very supportive of one another and the team would meet up approximately every three months, which Donna looked forward too.

A few years later and Donna was invited to take part in the Danish Open Swimming Championships in Copenhagen representing England. Now that was a very proud moment as I got to go over there too. She returned with only one medal, but lots of experience and in many respects, the medals were secondary and I always told Donna that no one could ask anymore than her best, if you give your best and don't achieve a medal, this should not be viewed as failure, far from it. Donnas swimming was improving beyond recognition and she very much wanted to join an able bodied swimming club that could take her to the next dimension, one that would really push her to her limits. Having done some investigation, I got Donna into Chester-Le-Street swimming club and this would prove an excellent move.

Although specific competitions would prove few and far between from an international perspective, Donna would remain an active member of the English Sports Association for People with Learning Difficulties and the England team for many years. We would travel all around the country to different venues and different competitions collecting a whole host of trophies and medals. She also made lots and lots of friends.

In 1996 Donna was nominated for a MacDonald's child of achievement award and travelled to London to meet stars from both sports and media at a gala event. She was presented with her award by Right Honourable John Major, at that time, Prime Minister. This seemed a million miles from the heartache of only eleven years earlier, when her precious life appeared to be slipping away from us.

However, in 1998, the incredible happened; Donna was approached by the head coach of the Great Britain Para Olympic team. He had been monitoring Donna's individual times for specific events and she had amaz-

ingly dragged herself into the reckoning for a place in the GB team due
to fly out to New Zealand for the World Swimming Championships in
Christchurch. The final place was between Donna and another young girl
and after much deliberation, Donna got the news she had been dreaming
of, the final place in the team was hers.

I was very proud to say the least the day her Great Britain track suit
arrived by post and she modelled the attire that evening. In the next couple
of months before she was due to leave England on that long journey to
New Zealand, Donna worked so very hard at training and even the local
television station arrived to feature her build up to the Championships.

The day came when Donna was due to meet up with the rest of the
team at London's Heathrow Airport. So early that morning Donna and
I set off to London by train and I remember at Durham train station, a
businessman came up to Donna and said he'd seen her on television a
couple of nights earlier and wished her all the luck for the forthcoming
competition. I was so proud, I felt seven foot tall, while Donna just stood
there and smiled.

It was not possible for me to journey to New Zealand with Donna;
however, I was kept informed by telephone of her progress in each and
every swim. She swam in the heats of the 100 meters breaststroke, her
favourite stroke and actually managed to make the final. The following
day the final was scheduled to take place, eight swimmers in total, Donna
would not only need a personal best in the event, she would need to sprout
wings as she had the slowest time of all the swimmers, importantly, just
getting to the final was an achievement in itself, but even more was to
come. In the final Donna did swim a personal best and finished seventh
overall, a fantastic feat.

Days later and Donna was picked to swim in both the 4 by 100 meters
medley relay and 4 x 100 meters freestyle relay. These races proved to be
very competitive, yet the Great Britain girl's team managed second place in
both events and subsequently, Donna came home with two silver medals
from the 1998 World Swimming Championships. I was the proudest dad
in the world and made it my business to tell everyone of Donna's achievement. I couldn't wait to see Donna on her return from New Zealand

and set about arranging a surprise party as a celebration with friends and relatives. Donna was at the top of her game and enjoying her swimming more than ever before. Some months later and a national event took place at Reading; naturally Donna would enter a handful of races. However, importantly, it was the successful relay team that would once again take the limelight during that event. On this occasion, not only did they win the event, they also smashed the world record at that time. To this day, that record hangs proudly on display in my study.

Significantly, both girls achieved much, only in different directions. They had huge potential to achieve great things at school, but like me, neither turned that ability into qualifications, but, as we have seen, it is never too late.

Admittedly, as a parent, I think there were times when the worry and fragility of Donna's illness that it became an overwhelming everyday concern.

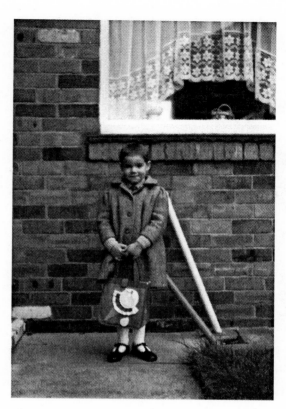

A poignant first day at school

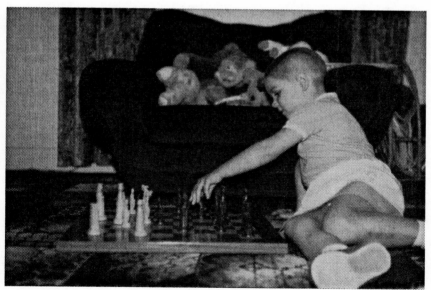

Checkmate.

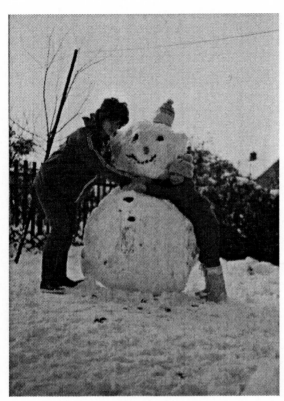

*Making a good recovery
and a great snowman.*

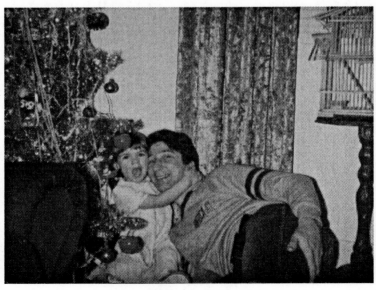

I love my Dad!

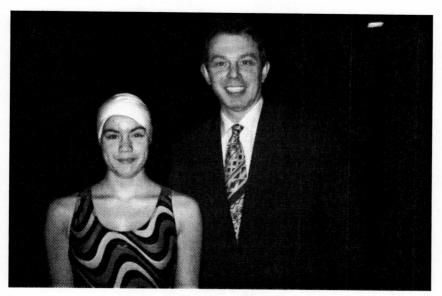

Donna impresses Tony Blair

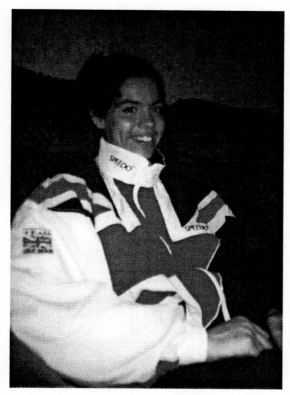

*Donna. Heading off
to New Zealand*

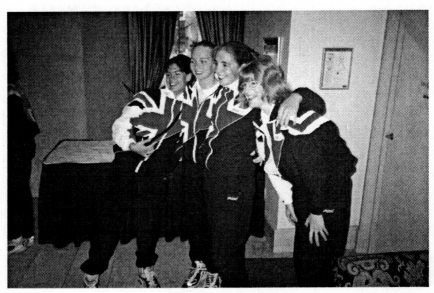

Donna and the silver medal team

Chapter Eleven

Eventually, the day came, when the results of the exams were due. I was up first thing in the morning drinking cups of coffee until I was buzzing with a caffeine induced high.

Looking In The Future

During the time when Donna had commenced her swimming career, life was at last, returning to normal. Therefore, I now had an important decision to make, a decision that would affect the rest of my life. I had, as has already been discussed, taken redundancy from my previous employment and as Donna was now doing very well albeit unexpectedly, then it was time to return to employment. The big question was what would I do? The answer was never in any doubt, nursing! I had developed a great respect and admiration for those who had nursed, encouraged and cajoled me through the real prospect of an early and premature death. I admired and respected the nurses who had more than just nursed Donna through a life-limiting disease. Nursing surely brings its own rewards, rewards that are worth more than any amount of money.

However, I had no qualifications to gain entry into the nursing profession and therefore, I returned to full time education for twelve months to gain the requisite qualifications that would allow me a new direction in life. Returning to education so long after leaving school proved difficult for me and I had to work especially hard to ensure I did not fall behind in my studies, still in a perverse sort of way it was enjoyable. I had taken five GCSE's and one 'A' level during that academic year. Yes, I could have stretched this over two years, but I wanted so desperately to begin my nursing career that one year it was to be.

Despite the ultimate need to gain the necessary pieces of paper showing the appropriate grades, getting into nursing would prove more difficult than I had anticipated. I was interviewed by three different nursing schools, Newcastle, Sunderland and Gateshead. Most importantly, at interview when asked why I wanted to enter nursing, I was completely honest about my cancer history and future aspirations. Unfortunately, even this far down the line and even the Health Service can demonstrate negativity and prejudice in respect to an understanding of cancer. Both Newcastle and Sunderland where impressed with my foresight and determination to make nursing a successful career and offered me a place there and then. Sadly, Gateshead and my first choice of venue to train felt that in view of my background, they could not offer me a place. Taking a place at Gateshead would have allowed me to work and hopefully, gain employment in my home town hospital, South Shields, the hospital which fourteen years earlier had made my cancer diagnosis.

Although disappointed, the belligerence of these nursing leaders left me confused but I was content to ignore their obstinacy and to accept a place to train at Newcastle. My immediate aim was to qualify and then work on ward 38 at Newcastle General where I had much of my treatment and then one day, return to my native South Shields to work in my home town hospital and give something back to the local community, specifically in cancer care. In May 1989 I commenced nurse training with pride and expectation.

Nurse training was hard work but very enjoyable and I was fortunate to train with a great group of student nurses, admittedly almost all females and I had the unenviable distinction of being the oldest student in the group and jokingly they never let me forget that point.

After an initial six weeks in the classroom we were all allocated a ward to spend ten weeks, gaining knowledge and experience of the nursing profession, while the training itself would take three years. My first ward was a surgical ward and I could not wait to start. However, I would soon have the enthusiastic wind knocked out of my sails. The ward was a busy unit dealing mostly with abdominal surgery, much of which was for malignant disease. In the first few days I looked after a little old chap who appreciated a chat as much as the nursing care required for his condition. Sadly, the nursing sister insisted that I met with her in her office; once in there she immediately laid the law down that I was getting too friendly with the patients. She insisted that I was there to learn not to befriend the patients. Well, I was more than taken aback and thought that she was pushing nursing back into the dark ages. Surely communication was identified as a fundamental aspect of care, so was it necessary to distance ourselves from the patient? I didn't think so, but hey, I was just a student nurse.

I think in many respects her approach spurred me on to hopefully, be a good nurse. Throughout my nursing career I met lots of nurses of varying degrees of aptitude and caring. I always remember the extremes of skills and the way in particular the minority would speak to and treat student nurses, without care or compassion. I concluded that if they could treat student nurse with such contempt then what was their actual hands on care like? It was those early days that made me determined not to follow the paths of those with a negative and dictatorial approach to their care, they were not good role models. I strongly believe that even today, nursing comes in for a lot of mostly unnecessary criticism, criticism that comes from the reputation of the minority of nurses who are not in the profession for the right reason. Unfortunately, it is this minority who the public recognise as the majority and that is not the case. Admittedly, there are nurses who do the profession a great disservice, but the vast majority are enthusiastic and dedicated to the cause.

I placed a great deal of endeavour on my theoretical work too as it was important to be able to underpin the practical skills with cognitive ability. My first piece of marked work was on 'Hodgkin's Disease' and most came from my own established knowledge and indeed reflected the lecturers comments, '*an obvious understanding and empathy of this condition*'. My pride endorsed the fact that this was the right career for me and even in those early days it was a pleasure and a privilege to be influencing the health of people dependent upon nurses and doctors in the health service. Even those individuals who were terminally ill, to be part of a team that improves their symptoms and makes their dying days peaceful and pain free was worth more than any salary could ever achieve.

In my second year of nurse training I actually got the opportunity to spend a placement (ten weeks) on ward 38. How would I feel nursing patients in the very same predicament that I'd been in thirteen years previous? My fear and apprehension was unfounded and that proved a very happy ward to work on. The staff, all aware of my previous illness were, without exception fully supportive of me and all the other student nurses allocated to the ward.

One of the Auxiliary nurses, Pat, was actually an Auxiliary when I was a patient and naturally we would reminisce about the years gone by. Being a nurse was a massive and steep learning curve; having worked in a shipyard previously, this was at the complete opposite end of the spectrum. Still, my mind was made up and my goal was to attain a job as a staff nurse on ward 38 once qualified. That would prove to be my motivation throughout some of the more difficult times. During my time on ward 38 I once again met up with Drs. Bozzino and Atkinson.

The staff were all aware of my previous diagnosis and subsequent treatment and remained very supportive. There were even specific times when the sister of the ward would approach me and ask if she could tell certain patients about my story and naturally, I never declined this request if it would benefit other individuals. On these occasions patients would often ask about the differences in treatment and how as an individual I coped with the sentence of cancer. Importantly, even in this honoured situation it would have been wrong of me to say '*I know what your going through*', because quite frankly, I didn't. Everyone is different as is their experience.

Working in the stressful environment that is cancer care causes many different kinds of pressures, pressures that need to be released and nurses are certainly well renowned for going out and enjoying themselves, it's called a release valve. However, the media reputation of promiscuity is not entirely deserved and is unwarranted. There were numerous times throughout my training and beyond that I would be invited out. Most often I felt that I had to decline these social occasions as my wife at the time would create merry hell and make all kinds of ridiculous accusations and insinuations such was her jealousy. Therefore, instead of allowing these situations to arise, I would simply make any excuse not to attend and even on the few occasions that I did go out with various nurses from different wards, I felt obliged to take my wife; at least it saved me from getting too much grief on my return home.

During nurse training, you would be allocated to a variety of different wards that would give the maximum amount of experience. I spent ten weeks on one of the paediatric wards and that gave a whole new dimension to nursing. It was not just the children who needed care; the parent's required psychological support and that presented a different challenge to your individual skills. Naturally during each and every placement the student nurse would be allocated a mentor, someone to supervise and support the student, someone to assess the skills you were to achieve on that placement. During those ten weeks, a difficult but enjoyable and an educative placement, I spent most of my time caring for a small boy aged two and getting to know his parents very well. His condition was uncontrollable epilepsy brought on by a condition which resulted in his skull being misshapen and which also affected his brain.

The child had spent most of his time in hospital trying, mostly in vain, to control the epilepsy and this reminded me very much of Donna. Some six weeks into my placement the Neurologist's were considering whether brain surgery would help improve his condition and it goes without saying that the decision was a very difficult one to take. It was at this moment in time that I made what I now consider to be a bad decision; I opted to ask if I could be present if and when the boy went to theatre.

Having reviewed the situation, the Neurologist's now decided to take the youngster to theatre and operate on his brain. The parents, although very anxious and concerned about the procedure, understandably, said that they felt a little better because I was going to be in theatre with him.

Things went well in the first couple of hours and went according to plan. Sadly, things quickly went rapidly down hill and he began to experience problems and subsequently he died in theatre. This was the most harrowing experience of my student days so far and not what I was expecting. How on earth could I now face the parents, as they had confidence in me being in theatre with their little boy, would they now blame me?

The Consultant Neurologist new that I had a good rapport with the parents and asked if I would accompany him to break the tragic news to them. I certainly did not feel as though I could refuse his request, but this was not something I had been trained for or was prepared to confront. Leaving the theatres, the parents were immediately outside and before we even spoke a word they new things had not gone to plan. To try and console parents in that situation, well there are simply no correct things to say and this was no exception, you cannot make that dreadful situation any easier for a parent. In fact, I struggled to maintain my own composure such was the extent of their unbearable distress. In fact, strangely, they were comforted by the fact that I'd been in theatre at the same time that he had died.

Later, once back on the ward I broke my heart, one of my colleagues was on the same ward as me and tried in vain to comfort me but to no avail. Life indeed, was so cruel. Where's the justification, the reasoning for the loss of an innocent life being needlessly wasted? To this day, I keep a photograph of the youngster at home in the study.

Life as a student nurse was extremely difficult, but also very enjoyable. Hand in hand with the difficult situations that one would face on the wards, there was also the exams and work that needed to be submitted and always it was a steep learning curve.

At last, during my third year I got the opportunity to return to ward 38 and this proved to be my future motivation. Without exception, the staff on the ward were very supportive and as I said, they new my background. I knew within the first few hours working on ward 38 in my last year, that once qualified, there was no other discipline I wanted to work, other than Oncology caring for individuals with different cancers and what's more, I wanted to work on ward 38. I felt that I had the passion, the empathy but also the dedication to deliver what is undoubtedly a difficult and unpredictable job, dealing with cancer patients and all of the physical and psychological problems they have. In addition, it was my contention that it would also allow me to give something back.

I now had another two student ward placements to go. None of these would match up to the satisfaction of dealing with cancer patients. Looking after patients receiving both chemotherapy, radiotherapy but also those in the terminal stages of their disease was the most satisfying occupation I had known.

I finished my penultimate placement and had only one more placement prior to the final examinations that would hopefully qualify me as a staff nurse, provided I passed the exams of course. The last ward placement was intended to consolidate your management experience and could have been anywhere. I now had a cunning plan, if I went to see the allocation officer and tell her a little of my history and also my desire to work in oncology, perhaps she'll be sympathetic and give me my last placement on ward 38. So I did exactly that and low and behold, the allocation officer was more than supportive. Subsequently, I had my last student placement on ward 38 and not only did this fulfil my needs, but the staff on there were superb, irrespective of my bias towards Oncology, they were a first class group of nurses and in hindsight an excellent team delivering a high standard of care. Even today I still see many of that team, even though there are only one or two left on ward 38, the rest, like me have moved to pastures new.

At the end of the ten weeks on ward 38 I prepared myself for the final weeks in class and then, our final exams. I was not good in exam situations but I wanted this qualification very badly. Everyone was full of their last placement and also their trepidations regarding the forthcoming examinations. All of the preparations complete, I knew that I could study no more and that it was now down to me, no one could do this for me. However, I had studied hard over the course of the three years and I was quietly confident.

Days before the exams and I got word that a junior staff nurse job would be coming up on ward 38 in the weeks after our exams and therefore, needless to say, I would eagerly await the advertisement for the post. The finals went brilliantly; there was even a question in there about cancer management that was ideal for me. However, like all exam situations I initially came out of the exam confident, but then began to sow my own seeds of doubt as I reminded myself as to the additional information that I thought I should have included. Sadly it would be weeks before the results were posted, what an anxiety provoking wait.

In the interim and the post on ward 38 was advertised and I immediately rang personnel for an application form. It arrived two days later and I sat down straight away to complete it. Once complete I took it personally to the personnel department at Newcastle General Hospital, I was taking no chances with the post. In the interim we were given teaching sessions on interview technique as most students were now seeking employment, in fact, one or two had already been interviewed for jobs and a few had been fortunate to get jobs.

Eventually, the day came, when the results of the exams were due. I was up first thing in the morning drinking cups of coffee till I was buzzing with a caffeine induced high. There he was walking down the path, the postman, pushing the letters through the letterbox and quickly rummaging through the pile of mail, I find the one I really want, it reads: *"I am pleased to tell you.."* I've done it; I had actually passed, what a relief, what joy. From being diagnosed with cancer seventeen years earlier, I am now a qualified nurse and determined to gain a future in cancer nursing.

Ten days later and a letter arrives which provides an added dimension to my thrust for a job. I have an interview for the post on ward 38. Days before the interview and I had spoken to as many people as possible regarding the potential interview questions. So many different permutations as to what might be asked; now I'm getting confused; now I'm starting to panic.

The day of the interview and I was as high as a kite. Sitting outside the interview room my heart was bumping so loudly that it was probably putting the other candidates off. Then, it's my turn to be grilled, as I stood, my legs turn to jelly and I wasn't sure if I could walk through the door. The interview panel were sitting there smiling and making it as easy as they possibly could. The questions started and I felt as if my tongue was covered with cotton wool, but eventually I got my answers out. It seems as though I was in there for hours on end before they release me from this persecution and promise to ring later that same day to inform the candidates of who has and has not got the job.

The remainder of the day and I could concentrate on nothing. Hours merge into hours before the phone finally rings with a well known voice on the other end; it's Marie, the sister from ward 38. She starts to tell me that I did very well in interview, while I'm thinking, just get to the bloody point will you. Then she says, "*We'd like to offer you the post on ward 38*". For once in my life I'm absolutely speechless, yet I mange to mumble something to Marie, thanking her for the offer. Later that night and I don't mind admitting that a bottle of 'Jim Beam' was emptied in celebration.

And so, things were eventually going as they should do and I could look forward to a new career as a staff nurse, working on a cancer ward.

Chapter Twelve

Wedding vows confirmed and we both walked back up the aisle to another Hawkwind track, this time the softer, ambient number, 'Lost Chronicles' from the Xenon Codex album.

Love In Space

The work on ward 38 was interesting and very demanding but also stressful; all the same I spent a very enjoyable seven and a half years there, learning a significant amount which would stand me in good stead as my cancer nursing career took flight. The team was a good one, made up of different characters who complimented and supported one another and also new of the importance of humour. Not only was it important that I consolidated my nurse training and gained some valuable experience, it was also important that I got the necessary educational additives that nursing demands.

During the first few months as a newly qualified staff nurse, I went back to college for one day each week and completed a teaching certificate. Teaching would prove an important component to my practice over the forthcoming years and remains so today, I do believe that it is important to share the knowledge we have learned with one another, no one has the exclusive right to information, it is one of the major ways to improve patient care, sharing knowledge and experience. Therefore, teaching is integral to the nursing profession. Of course what I do have and what I could not possibly share is my experience and knowledge as a patient, yes I can share my stories but that is still not the same as the cancer experience. It is, I believe, my best asset and the one that has enhanced my nursing practice most of all.

Mentorship is an important component of the nurse's armament, it allows the qualified nurse to pass on their expertise and knowledge to student nurses, equally, it allows the student to shadow the qualified nurse and learn from their tutelage. It is my belief that the knowledge I have accumulated does not belong to me alone, it has been gleaned from a variety of sources and therefore, I have an obligation to share it with others. During those very early days, one of the most important conversations I had with a student nurse and one that I repeated some two years ago was something that was influenced by my experience not as a staff nurse, but as a cancer patient. The student nurse who incidentally was very enthusiastic and determined to learn said to me during a busy early morning shift, *"Aren't cancer patients happy and well adjusted, they cope very well?"* Now this statement stuck in my mind and served as a good example of the stereotypical attitude of many individuals, qualified nurses alike. My response on this occasion was, *"remember, we only see these patient's when they are on the wards, we do not see them when they are at home"*. I think this is a very important point; nurses can go off duty at the end of a shift forgetting all about cancer care until the next day. In contrast, cancer patients do not have the opportunity to go off duty, they are permanently on duty, no matter where they are, or what time of the day it is. Often, the perception the cancer patient portrays is a brave face, coping with all that life throws at them and able to cope and carry on with life normally. But, how true is this perception? I would perhaps argue that in the main, this is a false illusion, not because they deliberately want to deceive health care professional, its simply that we do not realise the difficulties the cancer patient faces when away from the safety and security of a dedicated health care environment.

Of course, in those early days of my nursing career I still had much to learn about the discipline of nursing. On one afternoon, one of my patients, an elderly lady with terminal cancer was telling me about the times she enjoyed when she was a young girl. She began telling me that one of her favourite pastimes when she was a child was doing cartwheels for the benefit of her disabled brother. It was now that I got the bright idea of demonstrating my prowess at performing cartwheels and proceeded to cartwheel along the corridor, much to her delight. Unfortunately, it was exactly at this time that the departmental manager came onto the ward and demanded that I stop this stupidity and meet her in the office. Red faced, I met her in the office and was given a verbal rollicking. Now to me, I could justify my actions, there were no obstacles in my way and importantly it had given so much pleasure to this lady who was dying and what harm had it done, none that I could see. Sadly, the nurse manager didn't quite see or understand my rationale and I was instructed that this idiotic behaviour should stop forthwith. Only three days later and the lady who I had performed my acrobatics for sadly died, however the patient in the opposite bed had told me that the lady had told her family with great fondness about my show and which she truly appreciated.

Twelve months later and I had completed my teaching certificate, I was keen to continue with further education, but it had to be something that would have an impact on patient care. So, I applied for a scholarship from the North East Oncology Club and which would allow me to spend some time at Birmingham University to undertake a certificate in clinical hypnotherapy. Again, hypnotherapy would prove not only a huge benefit to my clinical practice but also my nursing career as a whole. Hypnotherapy remains an undervalued therapeutic tool that can not only enhance the cancer patient's well-being; it can also alleviate much of the debilitating side effects of treatment or indeed the symptoms of the dreaded disease itself. On completion of this certificate, I was one of only a handful of nurses practicing hypnotherapy in the health service in the UK. Significantly, over the forthcoming years, many patients would benefit from this complementary therapy that I was now using to great effect.

There are now many thousands of therapists's practising some form of complementary therapy and despite the growing success and popularity of these approaches there is little scientific evidence to support many of them, although some having more credibility than others? As early as 1994, research suggested that in excess of 70% of cancer patients had considered the use of complementary therapy at some point during their illness.

The key point I make here is that if someone you are aware of is considering any form of complementary therapy, remember, these approaches work hand in hand with conventional medicine, they are **not** alternatives. Equally importantly, when seeking out a reputable practitioner, and there is little doubt that that can be difficult, always ask about their qualifications and their background as sadly, there are many unscrupulous people out there quite prepared to take advantage of cancer patients.

Cancer patients are as varied and as different as the cancers that we treat, therefore, it is important that we seek out different and diverse treatment approaches. Almost on a daily basis, they present the health care professional with new challenges, but even so, it remains a pleasure and a privilege to be doing this work.

Working at Newcastle I was still seeing Dr. Bozzino or Dr. Atkinson on an annual basis for check ups, but also saw both on a regular basis in a professional capacity too. At one appointment, Dr. Bozzino decided to discharge me from his follow up clinics on the strict understanding that should I have any concerns, then I immediately contact him from a patient's perspective.

Much to my concern, some eighteen months later I would require his help again. I had begun to experience searing and unexpected pains in the head. Without warning and at any time of the day or night, it was like someone was inserting a red hot needle into my skull. The pain was only momentary but it was also excruciating and therefore, fearing the worst, I contacted Dr. Bozzino and confided in him the problem I was suffering. He wasn't quite sure what the problem was, but indicated that a malignant relapse could not be ruled out. Therefore, what he did was arrange an emergency brain CT scan.

Less than one week later I was contacted on the ward by the radiography department and asked to attend the following day, Dr. Bozzino had insisted that this examination was carried out sooner rather than later, yet the week's wait seemed like months and was accompanied by many sleepless nights and moments when mentally I would anticipate being told that my cancer had reared its ugly head again. To make matters worse I kept all of this to myself, I certainly did not feel that my wife was the best person to confide in and naturally, I did not want to worry my parents.

How would I cope with a relapse of my disease so far out from what I had anticipated was a cure? Many confusing thoughts went through my mind over those seven days and I do not mind confessing that at that juncture in time; I was terrified as to what the cause of these painful headaches could be; it was obvious what my greatest fear was. But, if it did prove to be a return of the cancer, what would my response be, I was well aware of the psychological struggle I had experienced years earlier. The closer the day came to having the CT scan and the more I convinced myself that this indeed was a recurrence!

Eventually, the scan was undertaken and thankfully, my fears proved unfounded and the scan showed no evidence of malignancy. Still, there must be a reason for this debilitating pain and so, Dr. Bozzino, confident that this was not a condition for him to address, referred me to a neurologist.

Later in the month I did see a neurologist who explained that what I was suffering from was a form of migraine, called 'ice pick' headaches. These were closely linked to stress and anxiety and I certainly had plenty of that at home. Still, I was relieved that this was nothing more sinister. Perhaps with the explanation of a cause, these 'ice pick' headaches would settle down.

At work, I had recently completed the Oncology course, a significantly important certificate aimed specifically at nurses looking after patients with cancer. Soon afterwards I was offered the opportunity to work as a higher grade staff nurse covering ward 37, predominantly female cancer patients and located downstairs below ward 38. This would be for a period of six months and this experience was supposed to stand me in good stead for the prospect of doing a higher grade staff nurse post when one became available on ward 38.

After eighteen months working in Oncology I was as happy as a sand boy, doing meaningful and fulfilling work and felt ready for a higher grade on a permanent basis. Importantly, I was encouraged by my colleagues that when the next higher grade came up, I should, and would apply. However, it would take a further eight months and three interviews later before I eventually secured a higher grade.

It never fails to amaze me the way that fate works. During the morning of a very busy shift on ward 38 I was met from the elevator by the feeble figure of a young man, his face pale and engraved with fear, I'd seen that fear in the mirror before. Unshaven that day, the beads of sweat stood to attention across his forehead as he introduced himself in a nervous voice, Simon*, he said. Unfortunately, such was the busy state of the ward that Friday morning I ushered him into the day room along with his brother and girlfriend, promising to return to them forthwith. Less than five minutes later I was summoned from the drugs trolley by Simon's brother. Understandably concerned, Simon's brother knew how important it was that Simon started some chemotherapy for his disease, a mediastinal Teritoma. However, Simon had other ideas and had decided that he was going to return home and forget about this chemotherapy business. Naturally, this situation took priority and I managed to find someone to take over the drug round in view of this situation.

I took Simon, his brother and pregnant girlfriend into the quiet room, the same quiet room that I had occupied with Sid some years earlier. I knew only too well this situation, but did not feel that I was out of my depth. Importantly, I could not just go in there and blurt out that I had also had cancer and knew what Simon was going through. Firstly, I did not have the faintest idea what was going through Simon's mind and secondly, I was going to be led by Simon. Given the privacy in this quiet area and the confirmation that he wanted his brother and girlfriend to come along in case he missed anything, Simon told me that he had heard so much about chemotherapy and knew he could not face the prospect of treatment. Simon was very close to tears but swallowed almost uncontrollably to keep these back and I have to admit I swallowed once or twice during that difficult encounter.

Simon acknowledged that his fears were founded around the horrendous stories of side effects that are often portrayed by the media generally and only serve to terrify future patients, leading them to expect or anticipate side effects that are not necessarily going to occur. My explanations of

* Name changed.

the potential side effects and the stressing that these were indeed potential side effects served to get our two way relationship off the ground.

Despite still being a novice staff nurse with not a great deal of counselling experience, I took a monumental decision, rightly or wrongly, to share some of my experiences with Simon, particularly my fears and concerns about treatment. Simon and I soon discovered that we had much in common, not least; we both came from South Shields. Furthermore, we shared a passion for rock music and Newcastle United Football Club and we both enjoyed the sport of kings (horse racing for the uninitiated), neither very successfully. But, most importantly, according to Simon, he was about to undertake the most frightening ordeal of his thirty two year existence – the commencement of chemotherapy for his cancer. Meanwhile, some sixteen years earlier I had embarked on that very same fearful and traumatic journey. This was to be our unique bonding!

So fate had played such a strange game with my life. Uncertainty and fear as a young man sitting in that quiet room aware that my life expectancy may be short, to sitting here now fulfilled and proud that I appeared to be helping someone in their battle against the physical and psychological onslaught of the cancer diagnosis.

For each and every procedure from now on, Simon would seek my thoughts and experiences on that particular matter. The medical and nursing staff were aware of our unique rapport and generally were supportive of the situation. Importantly, it needs to be pointed out that it is not my practice to tell all patients about my diagnosis and treatment experiences. On occasions, other staff members have asked my permission to narrate my situation to patients if they felt that that individual would benefit from hearing this and I have never declined that request as it may just help in some small way. In this instance with Simon, I knew instinctively, that it was the right thing to do, and so it proved!

Simon encountered many problems on this first admission, mainly recurrent infections that proved difficult to control and caused him to have an extended stay in hospital. Significantly, he suffered very few side effects from the chemotherapy treatment.

Sadly, over a period of some seven months in and out of hospital, Simon had set back after set back and control of his disease was never really attained. Infection followed infection and a bone marrow investigation revealed extensive infiltration, signifying progressive cancer. Simon and his girlfriend were spoken too by the Consultant and the Macmillan nurse and told of the fateful results. Simon was told face to face that he would not recover from this cancer. Strangely, although his girlfriend was understandably devastated, her eternal optimism now shattered, Simon appeared relieved and said that he always new this would happen. Sadly, Simon died at home only a few weeks later surrounded by the people who loved him.

I have no hesitation in identifying this incident as a positive one and worthy of inclusion. Yes, despite modern day advances in cancer care Simon did die. But, on so many occasions, he imparted to me how important our relationship was. Furthermore, at a time when, as a staff nurse, I was still consolidating my nurse training, this positive incident has had a great impact on my clinical practice, and I feel has moulded my practice today. Some few weeks after Simon's death I received the most fantastic letter from the family thanking me for the input into Simon's management. What greater thanks could there be?

So why do nurses working in the discipline of cancer services do what they do? Simply, because they are compassionate and committed, because they want to make a difference, they accept that it is a privilege to be involved with these patient's, yet the very nature of the disease and the fact that many patients will loose their battle equates to a difficult job. However, just because someone has a piece of paper, representing a diploma or degree, does not mean that they are any better at doing the job than the person who does not have that equivalent qualification, I sometimes think that far too much emphasis these days is given to those imperative pieces of parchment. Yes, of course education is vital in order that we can continue to grow and mature cognitively. Nurses caring for cancer patient's need empathy, commitment and above all, good communication skills to make a difference for the simple reason that if we fail our cancer patient's, then we also fail their family and that must not happen as it can leave a permanent psychological scar from that negative experience and results in a detraction from their quality of life.

After working on ward 38 for so long I felt that it was the time to search out my longer term aim, that of returning to South Tyneside where my original diagnosis had been made. Movement on ward 38 in respect to the more senior positions was almost non existent, even so and naturally, I was cautious as to moving on, I had such an unusual relationship with ward 38, first as a patient, but now as a staff nurse and part of a very successful and happy team and it proved to be a huge wrench leaving ward 38 such had been my unique relationship with the ward. Of course, it wouldn't be as straight forward as that, I would need substantially more and broader experience than I currently had. Therefore, after much deliberation, I had decided to apply for a post as manager (Charge Nurse) of a busy chemo-therapy day unit at Sunderland Royal Hospital.

Unknown to me and one of my colleagues off ward 38 had also applied for the position. Lorraine and I were very professional about this though and we wished each other the best of luck. Admittedly, Lorraine had more experience than I and also had a degree and although I was working towards mine, I did not actually have it. Low and behold and we both were short listed for the post and offered an interview along with other nurses from other hospitals.

I remember giving a very good interview and being told that we would be informed of the outcome the following day. We were both on duty that day and it was around mid morning when I took a phone call from the personnel officer at Sunderland. She asked to speak to Lorraine, which meant only one thing, she was being offered the job and this proved to be correct. Thirty minutes later the phone rang again, this time the personnel officer wanted me and informed me that I had not been successful. I congratulated Lorraine, but understandably, deep down I was disappointed. Still, this was the first senior post I'd applied for outside of Newcastle General Hospital and couldn't expect to get everything I would apply for; competition in nursing for such posts is high.

Then, you talk about fate taking an interventional hand. Seven days later and Lorraine had decided that her career would take a different direction. Therefore, she rang Sunderland Royal Hospital and retracted her acceptance of the senior position. Now, when she had told me this my feelings were a little subdued, Lorraine and I were not the only candidates, so would it be offered to someone else. If it was offered to me, would I accept being used as second best and want such a position having been overlooked in the first instance. That all important telephone call came within a few hours and the job was offered to me. I asked for the weekend to consider this and promised to call them back on the Monday. After much deliberation and soul searching, I decided that this was too much of an opportunity to decline. In addition, it was a significant stepping-stone towards my ultimate aim and I accepted this very prestigious and senior position.

Managing a department and group of staff was a significantly different proposition than anything I had previously experienced. Thankfully, I knew some of the visiting Consultants and this did help. In all honesty the small team were well experienced in the administration chemotherapy. In fact, I knew Paula, having done my teaching certificate with her some six years earlier; June I had met many years earlier when she had lived at the bottom of the street I had lived in and Donna had played with her little girl, Emma.

I was keen to start this exciting new role and test my own skills of management; my aspiration was to significantly influence patient care. Over the years in the position and after patient satisfaction surveys, senior management feedback, the views of the staff and most of all, the comments given from patients and carers, after three years and a half in that post I do feel I definitely achieved that goal. Many years after leaving, if I bumped into past patients or relatives the compliments were very kind and complimentary. The work was a mixture of oncology (solid tumours) and also haematology (blood borne disease, such as leukaemia's and lymphomas).

In all of the years of employment and socialising I had never had such a good friend and confidante as I did with June. From day one of my becoming Charge Nurse of the Chemotherapy Day Unit, we hit it off, in fact, we got on so well together that almost immediately; other nurses started rumouring that romantically we were an item, as only nurses do! In

A Love Affair With Cancer

fact, nothing could have been further from the truth, we were perceptive friends, she knew when I had a problem and needed to talk and I her; it was a very exciting and enjoyable time regarding work, but also a very difficult one as my marriage had recently failed and although I had attempted to keep this from my work and indeed the children, they had been aware of the domestic friction for some time. Donna was now eighteen, and I had to give serious consideration to my future and the direction it should take. Despite the fact that at that moment there was definitely no romance between June and I, there was certainly something drawing us together, at that moment in time it was not appropriate, perhaps the entity of fate was working here?

I had already confided in my sister Allyson, a full twelve years earlier on a trip her and I had made by train to Aberdeen that my marriage was not working. However, for the sake of the children, there was never a question of leaving so early in the lives of our young girls. They were completely innocent in the equation and in addition, they both deserved some stability in their lives. But yet neither did I tell my wife how unhappy I was in the marriage, to do so would have been a huge mistake and would have made life intolerable for both the girls and me. My decision would be to dissolve the marriage when Donna and her sister were old enough to acknowledge that sometimes, two people are just incompatible and have to go their separate ways.

My intention and desire to break up the marriage at the time that I did was filled with naivety. I had hoped that my wife and I would remain friends following the break up, particularly for the good of the girls, but sadly, this would be an impossible wish to attain, how stupid I was in making that assumption. The marriage had hit an irretrievable point, arguments were becoming a daily occurrence, but there was so much more than just arguments. It was a difficult scenario because the children were the innocent victims in this no win situation. Divorce proceedings would prove hostile and aggressive and naturally the children found the entire process very difficult, neither wanting to take sides. Further than this I do not want to be perceived as being vitriolic; therefore, enough said.

Thankfully, my friends and family were very supportive and aided my journey through the marriage break up. Soon after, I decided that I needed a new challenge and direction in my life and subsequently began searching for another job. Not long after this decision a position arose as a chemotherapy nurse specialist working for a private company in the community, was this the answer I was looking for? I was interviewed for the post and subsequently offered a position with the company, but in the ensuing months and in retrospect I would deduce that this was not the right move for me, particularly in those early days when the other chemotherapy nurses were very inexperienced and I felt misled and without clinical support, the onus of responsibility placed with me as the most experienced practitioner and I found some of the practices unacceptable. Staying there for a few years did broaden my experience and eventually the arrival of Karen would dramatically improve my feelings. I had worked with Karen at Newcastle some years earlier and she was a great asset and extremely knowledgeable, perhaps one of the most knowledgeable nurses I have worked with. Working in this role of course, would subsequently lead onto my ultimate dream and therefore I would again be thankful for my fate.

There is little doubt that at that moment in time, June would continue to be my best friend, our common bond, the break up of our respective marriages, and yet we had so much more than that, she was there when I needed a shoulder to cry upon and always ready to offer some rationale and pragmatic advice and this despite her own worries and troubles. I can't say when and I can't how, but at some point the close relationship changed from one of friendship to one of intimacy and romance, it was and remains the best thing that had happened to me in a long, long time. Love is the finest thing known to man and yet; in many instances it is spontaneous. June and I were no different and without a word being said between us, June and I fell in love and our relationship went from strength to strength and I think it is fair to say that we complimented each other to such a degree, that she knew my thoughts and I knew hers; at long last, I had found my soul mate.

Having lived with my mam now for almost twelve month I wanted to get my own place again, but finding something suitable may not be easy, in all honesty, I had no problems living with my mam, like my dad, I have a great relationship with my parents, but it was time to move on. Once again, fate would play its role. I had seen a seven bed roomed house for sale at a very reasonable price and although I didn't need that amount of bed rooms, I had to give it a viewing. The owner had decided to offer open viewing and along I went. Naturally, June came too. However, entering the house and it was plain to see that this enormous property was a very good price, yet required significant work, in addition, and importantly, it did not have a comfortable feel and subsequently I dismissed it from my options. However, leaving that house and June noticed that the dwelling next door was also on the market, a similar Victorian building with vacant possession. Therefore, I noted the estate agent and decided to call the next day. It turns out that this house had been empty for almost twelve month, once again; fate had intervened in my life.

Again, I took June and this time, her nine year old daughter, Sophie with me to view the potential home. The house had real character, built in 1896 and it had a fantastic feeling to it. Instinctively, I decided immediately to put in an offer that after some months of deliberating was accepted. There was lots of work to do but this was also an investment. Eventually, it was ready to move into. I had already asked June to move in with me, which she had agreed to do. In September 2000 we moved in together and during that first Christmas together I proposed to her, she had little hesitation with her response, and thankfully it was yes.

Not long after setting up home together we had the additional burden of extra lodgers, firstly Emma, June's eldest daughter needed a roof over her head and then Donna split from her boyfriend and had no one to turn too, nor anywhere to go and therefore her first choice was that of her dad. Therefore, quite naturally, she too moved in with June and I.

There is little doubt, that at times things were difficult but we never doubted our own resolve or relationship, which remained solid. Eventually, Emma would move in with her boyfriend and some time later would present us with a beautiful granddaughter, Courtney, my princess. It didn't stop there either. Donna too set up home with her boyfriend, Leon, although much to my dismay, this would be in London, still, as long as she was happy.

Amazingly and despite her previous treatment Donna would present us with a Grandson, Kieran. Now this is what life is all about, grandchildren. What's more, Courtney shares my passion for Hawkwind.

From an employment perspective, my dream came true in 2002 when an advert appeared for a Haematology Clinical Nurse Specialist at South Tyneside Hospital. There was little doubt that I would apply for this prestigious post, this was what I had yearned for. But, it's the same at every job application, you submit the completed form along with your curriculum vitae and then sit back and wait for the post. I was confident of getting an interview but not so confident of getting the job as there was sure to be other well qualified and experienced nurses expecting the same as me. A couple of weeks later and the postman delivered the letter I was waiting for, telling me of my interview date and the presentation I would be expected to deliver prior to the interview itself. For the next couple of weeks my head was inside of my books and the current legislation regarding haematology. Thankfully it all paid dividends, following the interview the telephone call I'd dreamed of came, *we'd like to offer you the post'.*

No sooner had I been told, I rang June at work to tell her the good news, next, I telephoned Karen, my manager who knew about my ambitions and explained that I would be tendering my notice, and she too was pleased for me. I couldn't wait to take up my new post, a post that I believe I was destined to fill. Since then, it has been a pleasure and a privilege to provide haematology nursing care at my hometown hospital, the hospital that had made my diagnosis way back in 1975.

My current role involves many different aspects of care including being involved with the Consultant Haematologist on a Tuesday morning, often breaking bad news diagnosis to patients and relatives. The strange thing about this clinic is that we use the very rooms where I, all those years earlier, received an abundance of chemotherapy, where I was told on more than one occasion that the treatment had failed, and the exact room where the junior doctor had attempted and failed to retrieve a bone marrow sample from my feeble chest. Ironically, as the haematology nurse specialist, one of my functions includes carrying out all bone marrow investigations. It is a strange entity fate, you cannot predict it, you can certainly tempt it but you cannot change it.

Working in the field of Haematology and dealing with individuals afflicted by the same cancers that both Donna and I had had is strange. How does it make me feel? Most definitely humble, but strangely at times guilty, guilty that I had survived when I had to acknowledge that not everyone does survive this feared disease. Most of all though, always privileged and honoured that I am in that position and influencing people's lives, hopefully making a positive difference to their quality of life. Only they can answer that. What I do know is that my own personal practice is heavily influenced by both Donnas and my own illness experiences.

Doing the job that I do, I inevitably see many people lose their personal battle against malignancy and that is very sad and very often difficult to accept. If I had a pound for every patient who I had been part of their care I'd be a rich man. Yet, in so many respects I am a very rich man, rich in the fact that I have and continue to play a part in the care of so many wonderful people, each one touching me in a different way. Forget about prizes and rewards in the health service, what better accolade can a nurse receive than the thanks and praise of the people they care for? It's all about patient satisfaction.

It would certainly be impossible to mention all of the individuals that I have had the privilege to be involved with, but one or two are significant. Stan, all the way out to Whitby. During my time delivering and administering chemotherapy to patients at home, he became more than a true friend. In addition to our professional relationship, he became a close confidante. In fact, his wife Angie, sons Ben and Lee, I would identify as part of my extended family.

John, a hard and dedicated business man, softened by the diagnosis of cancer, John was both fearful of the disease and yet put on a brave face, at the same time he and his wife became close friends. I was humbled to be able to help him in his final days by the use of hypnotherapy. Then there was Pat, one of life's stoical characters, what a privilege of leading, at her family's request, the funeral cortège on my motorbike, what an honour. And Carlo, a brilliant musician, an innovative drummer known by so many rock stars, I only new him for a short period of time, but his warm friendly approach to life generally made me feel as though he'd been known for many years, a giant among men.

Myra, we immediately found a connection and her ability to remain pragmatic and focussed is a tribute to her own ability of survival while her tenacity is just one of her many great assets. Doris, she honoured me by calling me her long lost son and at the same time she had such confidence in me to make her better that I feel as though I let her down when she sadly passed away, yet I was delighted when her family represented her at my wedding. More recently, young Sara, she was the same age as me when her cancer was diagnosed while she was given exactly the same diagnosis as was given to me some thirty years earlier and she has proved just as vulnerable as I was and yet her maturity is far greater than mine, innocence and naivety are her most endearing qualities. Her obvious difficulty confronting the psychological consequences of the condition reflected my own all those years earlier, her inability to deal and accept that she has a life threatening illness, yet I know and hope that she will do well.

In fact, I could easily fill a book with stories of courage and conviction from the many many patients I have had the pleasure to nurse and be part of their care, perhaps that could be my next book? So many fantastic people, the many brave individuals who have fought with dignity and pride against an illness that would ultimately claim their lives, but also those who continue in their fight against the most indiscriminate of conditions. I honour you all and thank each and every one for the participation in your care, I remember you all, and I hope I made a difference.

And what about when someone dies? We have two choices, either we can close our eyes and continue to be sad or we can open our eyes and remember them with fondness and recall the happy memories we have of them. I say that with sincerity and honesty and hope that it does not insult anyone, it is not intended too.

Inspirations just happen and I'm no different, at the age of forty-seven I had this sudden urge and desire to learn to ride a motorbike. In all of my years, I had been on the back of a bike twice but never ridden one, yet I now had this need to fulfil another dream. June was a little apprehensive, but if that was what I wanted, then she gave me her unconditional support. Subsequently, I contacted a local training school, did the required basic training, followed by the requisite written exam and then went on to do my full riding exam and passed at the second attempt. Now I needed a bike! But not just any bike, it had to have some credibility.

Subsequently, I bought myself a Daelim Daystar, a copy of the early Harley Indian; this would do for a few years till I got more and more experience, after which time the ultimate goal was of course, a Harley. For those who have not experienced it, there is not a better feeling than riding along the coast road, the wind passing through the helmet with the open road ahead. Freedom and pure escapism, a great rush.

And what of Hawkwind? Well, they continue to be a huge component in my life; in fact they will be until the day I die. In 2003 Hawkwind were headlining the 'Rock and Blues festival in Derbyshire, therefore as I had already decided on going I thought I'd take June and Sophie to see the mighty space rockers. Admittedly, they both enjoyed the bikes that were on display but sadly; neither of them was terribly impressed with Hawkwind. But in all honesty, it was not the best performance the band had ever given, but hey, a true fan takes the rough with the smooth. Over the years of following Hawkwind I have travelled to many corners of the land and met and kept in touch with many like-minded individuals. So much so that to other Hawk fans the length and breadth of the country I have become known as Hawklord of Shields.

Extremely content at work, Time rolled on for June and I as it does for everyone. Our years together have been good and although admittedly, there have been some difficult times to deal with, but never with our relationship; it remained and still is solid, rock solid and hand on heart, I can honestly say that we have never had a crossed word. On more than just an isolated occasion, June would ask, *"When are going to marry me"*, to which I would most often reply with flippancy, *"sometime"*.

But why was I always so flippant? Well, it had always been my intention to organise the wedding and then surprise her with a specific date. I had already agreed with Terry to be my best man, checked with important members of the family that they would be available to share this magic moment and so, in 2003 I booked the town hall for the following year, August 29th 2004 to be precise.

However, rather than surprise her in a restaurant by asking her to marry me and inviting her to join me at the town hall for the ceremony, which I knew she wouldn't appreciate, I had to think of an alternative approach. So therefore, when she suggested that we stayed in for my birthday and that we had the house to ourselves, then I thought that this would be the ideal moment to ask her to marry me. A candle lit evening, good food and a nice bottle of wine to enhance a wonderful occasion, I gave her a card with an invitation to her own wedding, including all of the arrangements and for once in her life June was actually speechless. Needless to say she accepted. That was a great night and will remain firmly embedded in our fond memories forever.

That was a particularly poignant moment for me too, why? Well, as I had arranged the wedding including the afternoon reception at a local Spanish 'Tapas' restaurant and a night time celebration at 'The Sea Hotel', I now told June that all she had to do was choose the music that she wanted to walk down the aisle too. June was startled at this request and felt strongly that she did not want to be walking down the aisle and suggested that I walk down instead. Jokingly, I retorted that if I walked down the aisle, then it would be to the sound of Hawkwind, astonishingly, June simply said, *"that's fine"*.

Now this got me thinking, was this such a bad idea anyway? I didn't think so. Hawkwind had supported me through some pretty bad times over the years, why shouldn't they support me at my wedding. As far as I was concerned, I could not think of anyone more important to be present at my wedding than the members of Hawkwind and with this arrangement they would be.

Subsequently, we agreed that June would sit at the front of the chambers with the guests and Terry and I would walk the aisle preceded by Courtney to the space rock music of Hawkwind, what a fantastic thought, what could be better?

The months ahead were filled with organising and arranging what would be a glorious occasion. On the day, the hall was filled with our guests ready and awaiting, not for the bride but for the groom, his best man and the flower girl. At precisely 1.00pm the registrar asked for quiet, and then, the sound system erupted to the sound of 'World of Tiers' from Hawkwind's Levitation album and Terry and I stepped confidently down the aisle with Courtney proudly leading the way, the distinct sound of Hawkwind echoing in the background.

We had planned and wrote much of the service ourselves and below is the opening extract that I would proudly read on behalf of the both of us and in the presence of our friends and family: -

In the presence of our friends and relatives, we have chosen to share our thoughts and promises.

On this most special of occasions, we promise to share our love, our friendship and our souls.

Like the stems of the climbing Jasmine, our love is entwined together forever and we promise to nurture that love to grow stronger daily.

As one body, we will share our emotions, our thoughts, our laughter and our tears.

In all that we do, we will trust, support and encourage each other.

Our promise to each other will be, although life is short, it is precious and therefore, we promise to assist one another to enjoy this life together.

When life proves difficult, we will half the burden by sharing the weight, and when life is good, we will double the enjoyment by being together.

Our loyalty is united, our bond unbreakable. And while we acknowledge and compliment our togetherness, we respect the others individuality.

This is our declaration to each other as you are our witness's.

Wedding vows confirmed and we both walked back up the aisle to another Hawkwind track, this time, the softer ambient number, 'Lost Chronicles' from the Xenon Codex album. This certainly was proving to be a day to remember, although it wasn't over yet.

At the reception and as tradition dictates, Terry read a number of wedding cards before he started his speech, but he saved one card until last. This final card he read out was, to me anyway, the best of all, it was a congratulations card from none other than the band, from the members of Hawkwind, signed by each and every one of them, and this was proving to be one of the best days of my life, Hawkwind had shared my wedding day as well as my illness and this was important to me. June was and is fully aware of the fact that Hawkwind are and remain an important component in my life, subsequently she had no hesitation in supporting my desire to share this special day with the band. Our night time party was something else again and a simple continuation of a brilliant celebration that will remain firmly embedded into the conscious and unconscious thoughts of us both forever.

The day after the wedding we jetted off to Santorini for a fantastic week on that beautiful Greek island.

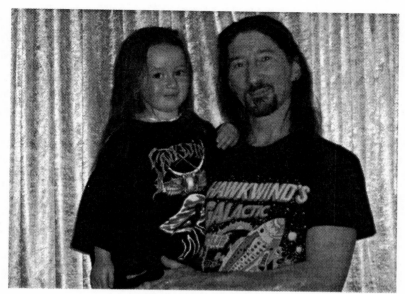

Courtney discovers Hawkwind, that's my girl

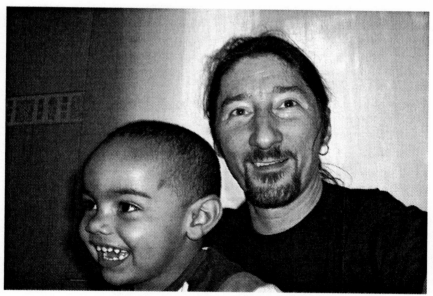

Kieran runs rings around Grandpa

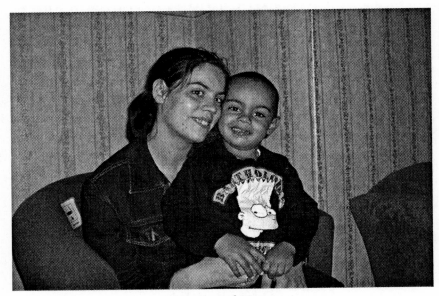

Donna and Kieran

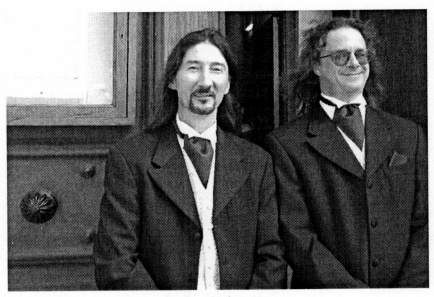

By far, the best man

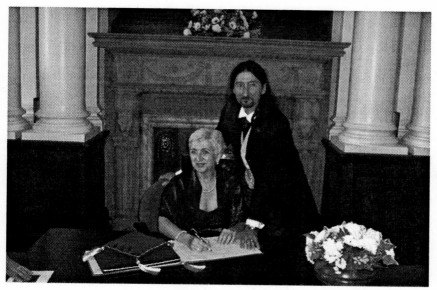

Sign here please

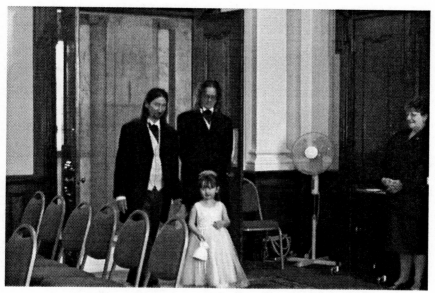

Proudly walking the aisle to the sound of Hawkwind

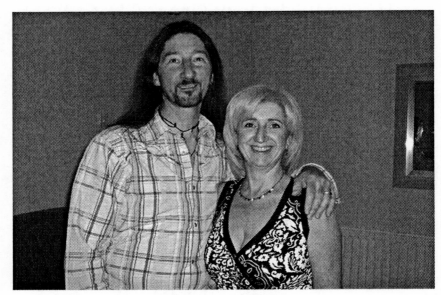

Ready for a night out

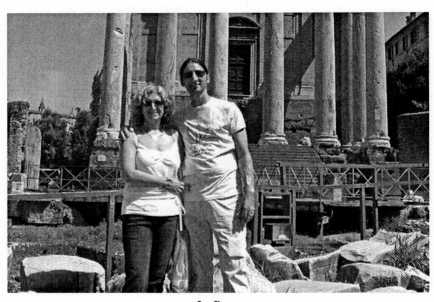

In Rome

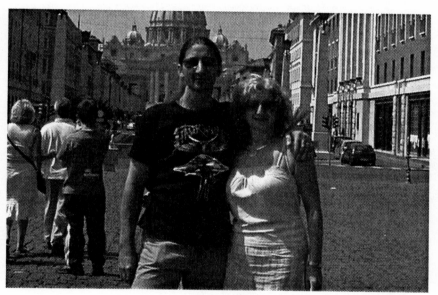

In Rome still

Chapter Thirteen

The cancer jigsaw is extremely complex and many pieces are still missing from the overall puzzle. We need all of those pieces to fit into place before we can solve the puzzle and see the whole picture.

Out Here We Are

Let's make one thing crystal clear, I'm not unique and neither am I special, many others have experienced the devastation that is cancer and undoubtedly, many more will follow on to do so in the future. But we must remember that a cancer diagnosis changes your life, it is a permanent attribute; it goes with you wherever you go and whatever life throws at you and although you learn to cope with it, it's just impossible to cast it away. Even though you may not think about it every solitary day, no matter what you do, it is always in the back of your mind and therefore, never far away. People who have had a cancer diagnosis learn to live with the most feared label that society is aware of. The experience will forever change your perception and personal philosophy.

It is probably, in my opinion, the greatest failing of the health care system today, the failure to address the long term psychological morbidity that goes hand in hand with a cancer diagnosis and, the relative demand for support that patients invariably need, particularly when they are no longer attending hospital on a regular basis. Give someone successful treatment for their malignancy and then tell them they are cured, however, the psychological baggage does not simply disappear because they have been cured. With every ache and pain experienced, the first thought to enter the mind is of a cancer revival, a relapse of the disease that you have tried and failed to put out of your mind and the untold fear that it elicits.

No scholar can define in a textbook the seriousness of a cancer diagnosis and all that it brings with it, unless they have been touched personally. Meanwhile, although healthcare professionals can certainly demonstrate empathy, they can only try to understand the true potency of cancer and it's ability to corrupt an individual's sanity, to influence emotions, to manipulate the mind and to elicit the greatest fear known to man. In my view, it remains a life changing experience of unparalleled equivalence.

Cancer is a word synonymous with fear and also sadly stigma and as the statistics tell us we all have a 1 in 3 chance of contracting cancer at some point in our lives, those same statistics don't tell us when or how to deal with it if or when it arises.

Does that mean that if one has already had cancer and subsequent successful treatment that one is therefore immune from those statistics? Well, I'm afraid not as we shall identify. Next to heart disease cancer is the biggest single killer in the world today and we are still no nearer an overall cure. Admittedly, enormous progress has been made in respect to treatment and also survival of many different specific cancers, particularly a condition called Hodgkin's lymphoma. From those days back in the early seventies, many would perish at the hands of this lymphoma and yet today, Hodgkin's disease is now most often linked to a cure.

However, as if to prove that cancer is a lifelong companion, more and more research is being published on the risks of developing cancer as a consequence of the very treatment that is used to treat the cancer in the first instance. As more and more individuals survive cancer we are starting to be able to piece together its long term effects. Although cancer survivors living thirty years plus following treatment remain in the minority, more and more individuals will attain that target in the coming years. Better detection of the disease and also more sophisticated investigations and improved drugs aimed at targeting cancer cells more specifically have helped improve the survival data for many cancers. We still need to carefully look at ways of supporting long-term survivors of societies most feared illness. The cancer jigsaw is complex and many pieces are still missing from the puzzle. We need all of those pieces before we can see the whole picture.

The published data in respect to developing cancer as result of the effects of treatment (Carcinogenisis) is rather ambiguous. Some data dismisses the risk while others claim that the risk is as small as 5% to as much as 60% depending on so many variables, including the type of cancer you had in the first instance, the type of treatment, age sex and much, much more. As yet, there is no definitive data to demonstrate this effect. In addition, there is also the theory that cancer is caused by a specific mutation. So, despite the very drugs known to be carcinogenic, then it may be that the same factors that caused the cancer in the first instance are the same influencing factors should a secondary cancer occur, so many unanswered questions, an incomplete jigsaw?

In retrospect, and importantly, as a patient, had I had this information some twenty-five years earlier, would I have gone ahead with the very treatment that I struggled to tolerate for so long? At the risk of sounding as though I'm sitting on the fence, this is not a question I can answer because I was never in that situation and therefore, I think you can only answer these questions when in that situation. Just like the person who says, "*If I had cancer, I'd..............*" To that person, and with respect, I say, until you're faced with that very situation you just do not know how you're going to react.

I discovered the details of secondary cancer as a result of my nursing career. At first, it hit me full in the face, as if I'd been hit by a centurion tank. For weeks I never slept and was uneasy with my discovery. So many questions streamed into my mind at the most inopportune moments, but more importantly, what can I do about it? Not a lot really other than to be aware of my own body and report anything of significance to the doctor and be aware of a healthy lifestyle as far as is possible.

There are no right or wrong answer with regards to whether patients about to commence treatment for cancer should be told of these risks in respect to long term side effects and yet, it is almost contradictory to deny people this knowledge, do they not have the right to be empowered to make the decision that is right for them. Paradoxically, is it right to burden someone with this kind information, they already have sufficient to deal with in the first instance. How many people might refuse the opportunity to be cured because of that potentially negligible risk of developing a secondary cancer many years later, if at all? Of course, and of equal importance, had I been told that information and then decided not to accept chemotherapy as a treatment modality, one thing is for certain, I would not be here now relaying my experiences to you. The ethical dilemma of Carcinogenisis will continue.

In my view, although this is always going to be in the back of ones mind, it is something that must not be dwelt upon, to do so, and you risk detracting from your own quality of life. If fate decides that course of action, then it will be addressed then, not until. Importantly, there is huge contradiction in the definitive risk associated with those individuals who have received chemotherapy and/or radiotherapy and the risk that those treatments carry in respect to secondary leukaemia's; however I do feel that it is necessary to highlight the fact that the risk is relative, remember that these leukaemia's are a rare occurrence in the first instance.

It is not my intention to discuss this issue any further as there are so many unknowns in the equation; equally, it is not my intention to scaremonger either. The issue is raised primarily from a patient's perspective. However, all of these facts are readily available on that wonderful medium we know as the Internet. The media have also been known to print articles on the very subject from time to time. Therefore, in many respects the health professional has an obligation to tell cancer patients about this risk and at least that way, we get the facts, not the fiction.

The media are responsible for much of the scare mongering in respect to cancer. Moreover, I am, and until they get it right, a big critic of the media generally. All too often we see negativity and sensationalisation regarding stories of cancer and details of those horrendous side effects of treatment. The problem with this portrayal is that it causes permanent damage in the minds of the innocent, causes heartache and unnecessary grief for those currently undergoing treatment and for those diagnosed with cancer and about to embark upon its treatment journey causing an expectation that those side effects, often graphically highlighted will definitely occur, instilling fear and trepidation into the very individuals about to receive the treatment. In my view this cannot be right, surely the media can appreciate that accurate reporting is not only their responsibility but also imperative to cancer patients. Now, I'm not saying that they should not report on public interest stories such as cancer; I'm simply asking that they report it with diligence and understanding of the need for accuracy. They never report on the thousands of patients who have chemotherapy and continue to work, the thousands of patients having treatment who do not experience side effects such has been the advancement in preventing the unwanted side effects with modern drugs. These common place stories do not sell newspapers or make for good television viewing and therefore, we seldom see these in the media. Subsequently, the media prefer to fuel the fear of society regarding malignant disease by simply endorsing the stigma that has become known as cancer.

The media also need to remember that cancer is not automatically a 'death sentence'. Today, the prognosis for many cancers is better than at any other time and advances are being made all of the time. New and improved drugs to help combat the unwanted side effects of treatment are now available and very effective, however, we should never ever underestimate the psychological scarring that is caused by a cancer diagnosis. And it is for all of us, the media included to address this issue.

Similarly, when new chemotherapy drugs are discovered, they should be reported with scientific awareness. Often, the headlines proclaim cure or new treatments for specific cancers. When these stories are examined in depth, the reporting is often way off target and wholly inaccurate. This in itself gives false hope to patients with the specific cancers sited in their features, and serves to demoralise individuals when they attend hospital to discuss these treatments only to be told that either they not suitable to their cancer or the drug mentioned is still in the trial phase and not actually available as a treatment at that time. Yes, the media do have an obligation to report new developments in cancer care but they also have an obligation to report it correctly. No one can imagine, me included, how it would feel if it had been read that a new wonder drug had been developed, only to be informed at hospital that this was not the case. We cannot play mind games with cancer patients as it can push them over the edge. Yes, the media have a responsibility to report new scientific discoveries regarding cancer treatments. But, their overriding responsibility should be to report them accurately and unfortunately, this is not always the situation.

In the same context, fertility issues raise a variety of concerns. We know which drugs cause infertility and therefore, there is a need to be careful with the selection of the drugs used for treatments, but also, individuals about to undergo chemotherapy need to be informed of the fertility risks. Sperm banking was never an option for me way back in 1975, but as the small number of longer term survivors increases we are beginning to realise that men can have a regeneration of their sperms, sometimes twenty plus years later.

It was the build up to Christmas, 1999 and it was the highest and lowest points in my life that came within weeks of each other. June had been feeling slightly under the weather over the previous few weeks, she had a suspicion as to what the cause was, but then, she had convinced herself that her suspicion was impossible. However, she returned home one night from work to tell me the news. I had the delight, the joy, and the ecstatic emotion of being told that she was indeed, pregnant and there is not a feeling like it in the world, an indescribable euphoria. What a high, what excitement, what anticipation and already my mind was filled with what we would prepare for our baby. December 14th was the date that is now indelibly imprinted in my mind and I was the happiest man on the planet and immediately began the planning process of what lay ahead. Will it be a boy or girl? What colour will we prepare the nursery? So many exciting questions and more importantly so many answers to look forward too.

Unfortunately, some twelve weeks later and we lost our baby to a miscarriage and I found that trauma harder to bear than the original cancer diagnosis I'd had to suffer myself. An emotional turmoil, no where to turn, tears followed tears, desperation and heartbreak, I had never known pain like it, my world had collapsed and my mind was filled with the thought of why life could be so cruel but I could not find an answer to that question. To this day, the memory of that ill fated event is as raw and emotive as the day it happened. My feelings and despair will forever remain a deep and personal secret. Inside my own mind, a deafening silence that would hide a million tears and a cascade of sadness lost in an unfulfilled paternal dream. Despite the support shown by our friends and relatives, no one could stem the heartbreak and utter emotional distress we were feeling. Significantly, Donna was an absolute rock during that very difficult time, ringing every night to offer support and a shoulder to cry upon, but no support could lessen the psychological destruction caused by that single experience. Cancer had attacked me with psychological turmoil and a physical adversity that was unprecedented in my inexperienced life, yet this trauma was inflicted so unexpectedly and the hurt was unexplainable, intolerable and enough to break my heart.

That experience is not something I would wish upon anyone and not one I'd want to repeat. However, until the day that I die, I will never give up the hope that one day, June and I will have a baby of our own as the tests done by our doctor conclusively showed that my sperms, although low, had regenerated.

Cancer has the ability to ensure that you reflect on so many aspects of life generally, to see life without the pressure of conforming to mainstream views, to evaluate all that life has to offer and make your own decisions about life. But, also reflect on your values and beliefs and for me personally, I was confused about the dilemma that is religion. I had to admit that religion is not only an important component to some people, it is also very powerful, but not for me. The views expressed in this chapter are solely my views and are influenced by the experiences of what you have read so far. Importantly they are not expressed to offend or insult anyone else's views or opinions but to rationalise why I believe what I do. In the same way that I do not judge anyone else on the grounds of religious belief, then equally I do not expect to be judged for the stance I take.

It's the ultimate question, a question we've all asked before and yet no one has ever, or probably will ever find the answer. The question? The meaning of life, where do we come from, why are we here, how did we get here and of course, what about God, does he or she exist? Phrase it how you wish, but it's a dilemma that has plagued each and every individual no matter what your cultural or religious beliefs are.

When an individual is faced with the diagnosis and subsequent treatment for cancer and the inevitable doubt about mortality, I am certain that almost all individuals would question their religious beliefs and that is quite healthy. Ultimately, there is one final decision to make, you either believe or you do not. In fact, I think for those who do continue to believe, and then there faith is probably strengthened in an ironic way. Mine, well, it went the way of scepticism. For me there were just far too many questions without answers. Yes, I was dealt a risky hand of cards of fate to play throughout life, I could accept that even if I faced the prospect of a very early death; Donna was blighted by this destructive disease and then was disabled by its legacy. Furthermore, when I witnessed what happens around the world with poverty and disease, the cruelty of life generally, wars fuelled by religion, then my mind was convinced that religion was simply a crutch. However, I must emphasize that it would never, ever be my position to criticise anyone else's views or opinions regarding religion, it is a personal choice based on experience.

Furthermore, it is my contention that to live your life in a respectable fashion (the so called, Christian lifestyle) and live life to the full respecting all others then you do not require the support of a religion. In theory, we are all made in the same vain and no one individual is any better than any other and as such we owe it to one another to respect each others individual values, yet, sadly, the world doesn't operate in that fashion, we only have to look about the world to realise that man is his own worst enemy when it comes to respecting one another. The world is filled with destitution and poverty, prejudices and hatred, very often founded around religious beliefs, bitter and savage wars have been a significant part of man's history yet these are most often initiated by religion. The Middle East is a perfect example, religious hatred destroying the essence of life as Jews and Arabs are in almost constant conflict, Catholics and Protestants have fought each other for decades in the name of religion, it happens all around the globe. But how can that be representative of religion, a so-called caring way of life? I just simply do not understand that! I suppose that's the weakness of mankind.

The earth has been around for billions of years and hundreds of Gods have been worshipped before the current one, who's to say that another won't take his or her place in the next millennium. There is no definitive proof that there is such a thing as God, yet people choose to believe it in hope and also fear and it is certainly not my place to criticise that hope or indeed fear. I have little doubt that there was such a person as Jesus, yet the bible is littered with contradiction and personally believe it has been grossly exaggerated over the years and much of this is to support the strength and hold the church has over people. Religion does not encourage individuals to ask the questions I pose here, quite the contrary.

Significantly, and prior to my own and indeed, Donna's illness, I did believe in a God, although I was never a fervent supporter. I guess like so many, it was a fear of denouncing a God in case there was such an entity and the risk of being denied at the end of life. However, in itself, that is a contradiction in terms and not the actions of a caring superior being. For many, me included, it is life experience that will mould personal or philo-sophical beliefs. If God is the creator of the earth, why is it that the planet is so unpredictable? Earthquakes, hurricanes, tsunamis and unpredictable weather, usually inflicted on third world countries. That's a caring creator? Not in my view, and ironically, these elements that are so destructive to innocent life are referred too as 'Acts of God'. All around the world there are bloody and oppressive wars, most often in the name of religion, and I therefore concluded, in my opinion, there is no definitive evidence to endorse a God.

I believe that Religion and hypocrisy go hand in hand. Take for example the extremely harrowing and sad and importantly catastrophic earthquake that took place in Asia recently, the comments from one of the religious leaders was offensive and a contradiction to the ethos of religion, no matter which faith you follow. A Mullah argued that "the earthquake was a punishment from Allah" (The Daily Telegraph, Saturday October 15, 2005) now if that is not misguided and out of touch with the true essence of religion well, I'm not sure what is.

It is my understanding that religion is supposed to bring people together with a forgiving and compassionate ethos, yet the world over; religion proves divisive, confrontational and causes segregation across all of the different sects and beliefs. Shouldn't all religious believers be united and worship the same God or is that too simplistic?

Science can now explain and more importantly, prove the origins, the evolution of the universe, formed by the merging of gases and minerals billions of years ago. Physics explains that within the universe there are many hundreds of different galaxies and many of these may be capable of supporting life.

To me, religion simply does not stand up to scrutiny and analysis. It is my philosophy that we should treat others with the same respect that we would expect for ourselves and despite our differences in respect to religious, cultural or political beliefs. Remember, we all have an opinion, we should not therefore judge others because their views are different to our own, essentially, that really is one of the component's that makes this country great. Life is too short for any approach other than mutual respect. Enjoy it while you can, for if you don't, one day, it'll be too late.

That said, I do not intend to sound 'holier than thou' but significantly, I do not believe that I am judgemental, I have my own views and opinions on many things as we all do; and neither do I think that any of my actions over the years have been taken in a deliberate attempt to hurt anyone, I firmly believe that we are all entitled to the freedom of speech we enjoy without fear of retribution. I live each and every day the only way I know, grateful for every day as it comes around knowing that I am fortunate to be alive and passionate about my music, my work and my family life; I love my wife and look forward to the future ahead, unsure as to what it holds. Equally, my views expressed in this chronicle are not intended to upset or offend; they truly represent the way in which cancer has manipulated my thought processes and ideals.

Never look back on your life unless you are prepared to smile and be reflective, never look forward unless you can dream. We all need dreams and we all need hope. Life is a difficult entity, but it's there to be enjoyed no matter what.

Chapter Fourteen

Then, at the annual Hawkwind Christmas concert at London's Astoria in December, I got an invite to the band's after show party and eventually, after a thirty three year wait, I met and chatted with the man who for all that time had been my best friend, yet in all of that time I had never had the privilege of meeting, Dave Brock, leader of Hawkwind.

Take Me To Your Leader

I t started with my musical discovery, with none other than Hawkwind, but then led to a sick role as a cancer patient and an associated psychological distress eventually followed by a subsequent personal maturity, but also a realisation and sense of what life was really all about, its beauty and innocence, its good points and also the bad aspects of life too, a character building experience matched by no other. But also an acknowledgement that as a cancer patient a coping mechanism was essential, at least for me anyhow, everyone copes in difference ways, Hawkwind proved to be my coping mechanism and without them I would have struggled. Equally, and as importantly, my family were my support mechanism.

Throughout the whole journey, I had discovered myself, someone I had not known until that moment. It then continued with the harsh and abrasive reality of being the parent of a child struck down by cancer, the destructive essence of coming close to losing your only child to the predatory enemy of leukaemia, the desperation and helplessness that only a parent can know. The joy and gratitude of survivorship from both perspectives and then the role of student nurse and the ascendancy to Haematology Nurse Specialist, a unique and most importantly, privileged rotation.

Today, my passion for a good practical joke is as strong as anyone else and I'm the first to acknowledge that I'm as daft as they come and for that, I make no apologise, I love life and all that it has to offer, but also all of the challenges that it continues to present and much of this is down to my experience as a cancer patient. But my life is not, by any stretch of the imagination over yet, it continues today, as the ever youthful Hawkwind still actively tour on a regular basis, fuelling my travels around the country. From travelling to a gig in Belfast to the next in Manchester, from Newcastle to London and everywhere between, Hawkwind remain a significant component in my life, their inventive edge remains as sharp as ever, if not sharper. Significantly, I'm supported in my endeavours to follow and support Hawkwind by my wonderful wife, June.

And so, from 1975 to the present day, so many life changing events have occurred and in many respects, it has been and continues to be a fantastic journey, unmatched and unrivalled by any work of fiction and yet, the realism of the cancer experience has impacted upon my own personal beliefs and philosophy changing my outlook on life forever. But, I've now travelled full circle, and, although the future can never be seen as absolutely certain, my fate is already mapped out in front of me. What further surprises will it have in store? Who knows. I certainly don't.

Time stands still for no man and there is one important question that never goes away, particularly as the years march on, a question that frequently navigates my deep inner thoughts, even after thirty years and despite my own pragmatism, or my own logical thought process's, the question remains...

Will it ever come back?

Today, when alongside the Consultant Haematologist and we see patients in the very same cubicle where I endured that bone marrow investigation over a quarter of a century ago and then went on to receive so much intravenous toxic poison, my thoughts occasionally wonder, will I ever be in there again as a patient?

Perhaps it's because of the work I do or possibly it is due to my new sense of security and happiness I have found with June that this question is now more prominent in my mind than ever before. Yet, there are aspects of my life that remain sad, but perhaps one day that sadness will also be resolved, I hope so.

Today, the prognosis for lymphoma is far more favourable than way back in the seventies, however, we should remember it can, and still does claim lives. The treatment itself has become so much more refined and the side effects profile is far better than ever before, yet no matter, the navigation through chemotherapy remains a difficult one, both physically and without fear of contradiction, psychologically. That said I do not seek to underestimate the severity of a cancer diagnosis or even the debilitating effects of any of its necessary treatments given today. Unfortunately, even in the modern health service today, there remains so much stigma and misconception around cancer and its valuable treatments, so many individuals expect or anticipate nothing but negativity and debilitating side effects, when in reality, the dosages of drugs are calculated so much more carefully, which limit the toxicities. The drugs available to prevent nausea and vomiting are so much more efficacious than ever before and the support from health care professionals is now well established. Written information about all aspects of cancer management is accessible to all cancer patients should they require it, something unheard of thirty years ago? Providing the written information allows individuals to make informed decisions, but also to satisfy their need for at least some control.

Significantly, a cancer diagnosis is an individual experience; it affects each and every one of us in a different way. But, the one solitary similarity, the single unification is that a diagnosis changes your perception of life forever. Without doubt in my opinion, the cancer journey that I undertook all those years ago was not only a difficult road to trek, it permitted me to mature personally, to respect life and improve my own quality of life through reflection and appreciation. Furthermore, the traumatic pains of witnessing Donna suffer at the hands of an impartial disease, indiscriminate in its choice of person, left me bewildered and helpless to help my own child. But, being able, with Donna's help to adjust and learn to live with her disease and take from it positivism and that a cancer diagnosis does not automatically mean a death sentence. Therefore, it does not have to be a negative experience, despite the difficulty of coming to terms with it or the hardship of living with cancer, more support than ever before is available. Importantly, I fully appreciate that not everyone diagnosed with a cancer diagnosis will be as fortunate as Donna and I were, but hopefully, one day they will be.

When the cancer patient has completed treatment he or she is seen at regular intervals in clinic. The longer they stay in remission, the greater the time interval between clinics visits. Then, the patient suddenly feels more vulnerable with an associated absence of support. From the intensity of regular visits for treatment to the occasional visit for review. Cancer patient's, particularly long term survivors are entitled to more support than is currently available. Today, more and more individuals survive the cancer experience, an acknowledgement to the advances science has made in respect to treatment approaches. As the survival curve becomes more acute then the health service needs to make provision for the psychological care requirements of these survivors.

Communication is at the heart of psychological care and to deliver that fundamental care, health care professionals must learn to develop closer relationships with cancer patients. Following on from my diagnosis, it was clear that many nurses and doctors would actively distance themselves from cancer patients in fear of being confronted by their own uncertainty as to how they should respond. However, when Donna was diagnosed, the approach, although still far from perfect was so much better than my experience in the seventies. Health care professionals, particularly the nurses would often communicate with honesty and sincerity no matter what question was asked, whether that questions was asked by a child or a parent. Cancer patients deserve to be supported through what is ultimately a challenge to their very existence; the most appropriate support health care providers can offer is through good communication that can increase the satisfaction of care and provide a trusting and emotional relationship.

Survivorship is sometimes just as difficult to deal with as the actual diagnosis, there is a difficulty predicting what the future holds as cancer is such an unpredictable entity. The emotional fear that it evokes does not disappear, even after the all clear has been given and in my opinion, psychological morbidity can debilitate an individual in the same way and occasionally worse that the physical symptoms activated by the cancer and its unforgiving treatment. Therefore, I would leave you with one final thought, if we do not treat each and every patient psychologically, is it worth treating him or her at all? Psychological support is such an important component of care for any cancer patient, that health care professionals ignore it at their peril. Psychological care is a life long need for cancer patients; it needs to be a core component of the planned care pathway.

Like all other individuals who's life has been affected by a cancer diagnosis, my journey was a unique one and yet it touched more than just my life, my diagnosis was not mine alone, it belonged to everyone important to me and it touched them almost as much as it touched me.

From those early days of my diagnosis and indeed, soon afterwards, it was thought that the entity that is cancer would terminate my existence proving a totally destructive experience. The unequalled fear of losing Donna was an experience that simple words could never explain. Yet, there is no doubt, that my personal profile has been enhanced by the positive experience of a cancer diagnosis, as the parent of a cancer child and despite the fact that June, the love of my life, is my number one passion, throughout my cancer journey and beyond, during my darkest moments, Hawkwind were a constant passion just as my family were a constant support.

So what has been my magical formula in life? Well naturally, there is not one single factor or component that can claim to be the reason I overcame cancer. For me as an individual there were many reasons, not least of these was the support and love from my family and despite their attempts at misguided, but well intention collusion I would not be here today without them. The inspiration and time held dreams that Hawkwind gave me without taking anything in return. The doctors and nurses whose dedication and commitment to the cause was unswerving. My friends who became an extension to my family, looking out for me and accepting and cajoling me through some dark moments, you all know who you are. My positive mental attitude which focussed my attention on the fact that this was a life-threatening illness, and yet, there were times when I was emotionally unstable and bereft of happiness as the positive mentality proved an impossible direction to steer. But almost paradoxically, I felt that the unhappiness and depression was an important release valve. Despite the urges of so many to insist and plead that I maintained the 'think positive' attitude, it is sometimes easier said than done and I firmly believe that cancer patients, are entitled to feel sorry for themselves from time to time. Significantly, I'm also sure that most, if not all would agree that a 'positive mental attitude' is a major ingredient when it comes to fighting cancer.

In contrast, Donna's illness was so much harder to accept and contend with. My helplessness and sense of inadequacy when she needed me most was enormous, not knowing at that moment that what she was receiving throughout her cancer experience was something that could not be bought, love! A transference of a sense of being wanted, being special and unique as all children are. Strangely, her reciprocation to us as parents gave her a purpose in life.

Everyone copes differently with a cancer diagnosis, there is no one element that is above all others and my story is no different in that respect and as such it is not intended to be prescriptive or a specific guide to others. It has allowed me to appreciate what many take for granted, to reflect on my own mistakes and there have been many. Most importantly, it allowed me to discover myself and to live life to the full and enjoy each and every day as it happens. One day will be my last and therefore, I do not want to have any regrets about how I lived. Even so, like everyone, I still have dreams, I still dream of being part of the Hawkwind experience more closely, perhaps being part of the road crew for their next tour or being with them in the studio when they lay down the tracks for the next album, life is made up of dreams.

Take from my experience whatever you choose, criticise it where you feel necessary, but always remember that this was my experience of cancer as an individual and a parent and I truly believe it has made me the person I am today, that being a better person, philosophical, caring and determined to make a difference somewhere.

Moreover, when ultimately my time is at an end on this plane, my one wish is that I am heralded into the funeral service to the sound of 'Out Here We Are' a modern day Hawkwind masterpiece. A fitting tribute to what, in my opinion, has been a fulfilling existence.

All of the chapter titles in this book are named after Hawkwind songs, but that's probably no surprise to anyone, while I have tried to choose specific titles that I could link to specific episodes of my life. Hawkwind are such a huge part of my life that one day (although hopefully not for a long time to come) they will share my funeral celebrations too.

2004 was a significant year; in August I re-married and walked down the aisle to the sound of Hawkwind. Then, at the annual Hawkwind Christmas concert at London's Astoria in December, I got an invite to the band's after show party and eventually, after a thirty three year wait, I met and chatted with the man who for all that time had been my best friend, yet in all of that time I had never had the privilege of meeting, Dave Brock, leader of Hawkwind.

Cancer remains a modern day stigma, sensationalised by the media to fuel the fear of many, but it doesn't have to be that way. For me, it has moulded me as a person, it has shaped my very future, while equally importantly, it has manipulated my life philosophy, and it directed my career path to new and proud heights. I can see a different side of my character, I can appreciate an in depth dimension to the things that make up the everyday world and I have a commitment and passion for music, a dedication to my family and a respect to all others. Cancer took my innocence and moulded it into maturity, belief and respect, yes; it truly is and will remain 'a love affair with cancer'.

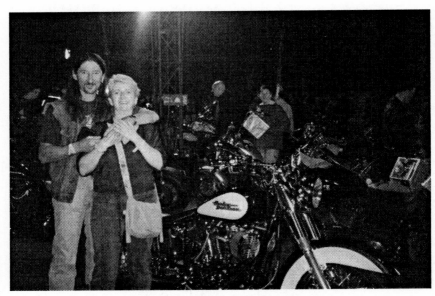

Rock and Blues festival 2003

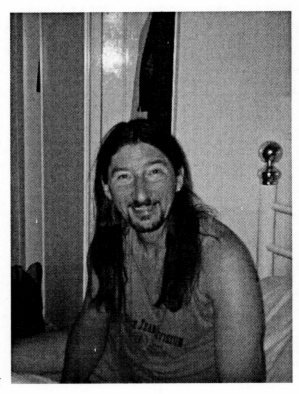

Just chilling

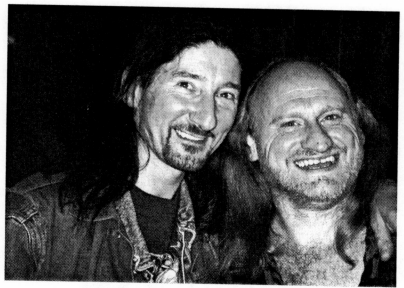

With Alan Davey, Hawkwind, Bass guitar

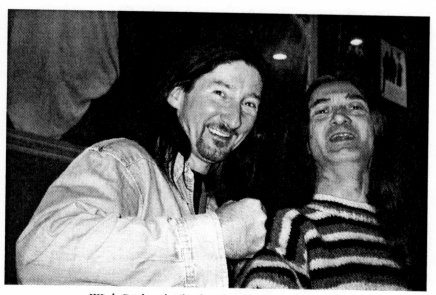

With Richard Chadwick, Hawkwind, drums

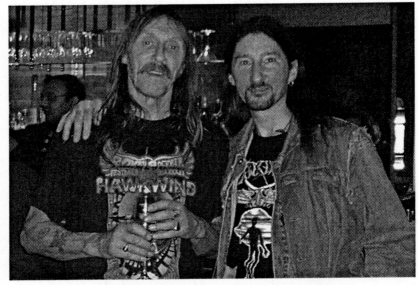

Finally, I meet Dave Brock after 30 years waiting

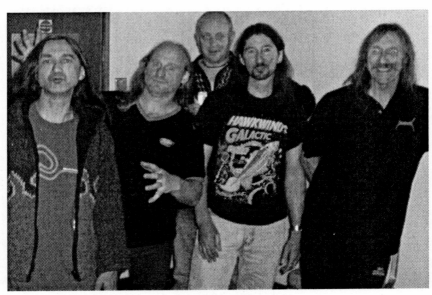

Croyden, 2005

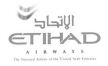

— Coral Menu —
heathrow – abu dhabi

tandoori chicken and pasta salad

saffron and yoghurt zorbian chicken, white rice, vegetable saloona

arabian lamb leg tagine in moroccan spices, vegetable couscous

tomato and parmesan cheese risotto, forest mushroom ragout

arabic date cheesecake, cardamom vanilla anglaise

cheese

tea and coffee

hot chocolate

refreshment will be offered before landing

"bar service"
wines: white and red
spirits: scotch - ballantine's, gin - gordon's
vodka - smirnoff red, bacardi rum
beers: heineken, bitburger and amstel light
liqueurs: selection of liqueurs
soft drinks
carbonated and still water
selection of juice

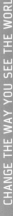

CHANGE THE WAY YOU SEE THE WORLD

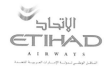

النــاقل الوطنــي لدولــة الإمــارات العربيــة المتحــدة

—— **قائمة المرجان** ——
هـيـثـرو ـ أبـوظـبـي

دجاج تندوري و سلطة باستا

دجاج ذوربيان باللبن والزعفران، أرز أبيض، صالونه خضار

طاجين برجل الضأن بالبهارات المغربية، خضار بالكُسكُسي

طبق أرز ريسوتو بالطماطم وجبنة البارميسان، يخنة فطر فورست

كعكة جبنة بالتمر العربي، فانيلا إنجليزية بالهال

جــبــنــة

شاي وقهوة

شوكولا ساخنة

سوف نقدّم لكم وجبة خفيفة قبل الهبوط

"خدمة المشروبات"
المرطبات
كوكا كولا، كوكا كولا (لايت)
سبرايت، سبرايت (لايت) وجنجر آيل
المياه الغازية : صودا ، تونيك ، بيرييه
تشكيلة من العصير
مياه معدنية طبيعية

My Final Thoughts

"There is so much trouble and disagreement in the world today, for whatever reason. However, in the greater scheme of things, life is so short and precious. Subsequently, I sincerely believe that if we acknowledge our differences and treat each other with the same respect that we would expect for ourselves, and then the world would be a better place, simply by appreciating one another.

Life for each and every one of us is unique, unknown in its ultimate duration and yet so many individuals take it for granted. Life is not a rehearsal, it is for living, it is a once only opportunity to enjoy, to manipulate for your own benefit. The future is uncertain; no one knows what lies ahead, what fate has planned. Therefore, live life to the full, enjoy it as if each day were your last, one day it will be and you should have no regrets to leave behind as a legacy.

Life is precious, a wonderful entity, an entity to be enjoyed to the full. Surviving cancer and witnessing Donna overcome the burden of leukaemia allowed me to reflect on so many different components in life, to see why I should enjoy the moment instead of planning for the next. It does not just have to be a cancer experience that changes people, it does not need a cancer diagnosis to appreciate life, to realise how precious it truly is.

No one person can deny anyone else the opportunity to enjoy life to the best of their ability, but it remains your responsibility to do so".

Printed in the United Kingdom
by Lightning Source UK Ltd.
119336UK00001B/215